YOUR
NEW
PRIME

YOUR NEW PRIME

30 Days to Better Sex, Eternal Strength,
and a Kick-Ass Life after 40

CRAIG COOPER

with Andrew Heffernan

HARPER WAVE

An Imprint of HarperCollins*Publishers*

This book contains advice and information relating to health care. It is not intended to replace medical advice and should be used to supplement rather than replace regular care by your doctor. It is recommended that you seek your physician's advice before embarking on any medical program or treatment. All efforts have been made to assure the accuracy of the information contained in this book as of the date of publication. The publisher and the author disclaim liability for any medical outcomes that may occur as a result of applying the methods suggested in this book.

HarperCollins books may be purchased for educational, business, or sales promotional use. For information, please e-mail the Special Markets Department at SPsales@harpercollins.com.

FIRST EDITION

Designed by Kris Tobiassen of Matchbook Digital

Photographs copyright © Kremer Johnson Photography

Library of Congress Cataloging-in-Publication Data

Cooper, Craig
  Your new prime : 30 days to better sex, eternal strength, and a kick-ass life after 40 / Craig Cooper with Andrew Heffernan.—First edition.
    pages cm
  ISBN 978-0-06-235324-5 (hardback)—ISBN 978-0-06-235325-2 (trade paperback)—ISBN 978-0-06-235326-9 (ebook) 1. Men—Health and hygiene. 2. Physical fitness for men. 3. Men—Nutrition. 4. Testosterone—Physiological effect. I. Heffernan, Andrew. II. Title.
  RA777.8C66 2015
  613'.0423—dc23
                                  2015012774

15 16 17 18 19 OV/RRD 10 9 8 7 6 5 4 3 2 1

To Maria, my partner in life and business for thirty-five years.
And to Montana and Lauren, who are all the reasons I need to stay healthy.

Nothing in this world can take the place of persistence. Talent will not; nothing is more common than unsuccessful men with talent. Genius will not; unrewarded genius is almost a proverb. Education will not; the world is full of educated derelicts. Persistence and determination alone are omnipotent.

—CALVIN COOLIDGE

CONTENTS

PART I: TOPPING OFF YOUR T TANK: OPTIMIZING YOUR LIFE FORCE

PART II: FUEL AND FLAME: NUTRITION AND EXERCISE

PART III: SEX, STRESS, AND OTHER CONFUSING STUFF: TUNING UP YOUR BRAIN—AND YOUR BALLS— FOR THE LONG GAME

PREFACE

TWO ROADS

> For the meaning of life differs from man to man, from day to day and from hour to hour. What matters, therefore, is not the meaning of life in general but rather the specific meaning of a person's life at a given moment.
> —Viktor E. Frankl, *Man's Search for Meaning*

What is the meaning of your life right now?

This may seem like an odd question. But as men in our middle years, we all wrestle with it. Who are we? What is this phase of our lives all about? And what kind of life do we want going forward?

Back in our twenties, thirties, and early forties, life's pursuits seemed a lot clearer. A sense of identity, belonging, and achievement. Some headway toward our dreams: A successful career, a loving partner, financial freedom, a nice house, great kids. Adventure. Fulfillment. Travel. But for a lot of men, the life map we created at an early age got a lot fuzzier as we approached forty. If anyone had asked us back then how we envisioned our post-forty lives, we probably would have shrugged and responded, "I'll be rich and retired," or "I'll have it all figured out by then," or "I'll have a Nobel Prize, an Academy Award, a Pulitzer, and my face on the cover of *Fortune*." Or maybe we didn't even think we'd make it past forty.

Now that we're here, though, the view is a little different. The checklist is out, and we're tallying up the wins and losses: Are we as successful as we'd hoped? Do our partners love us unquestionably? Have our children turned out the way we envisioned? Are we kings of the castle, masters of our domain? Are we performing at the level we want, in all the areas that matter—physical, sexual, and mental?

I don't know a single guy—no matter how successful—who has let himself off the hook in this compulsory half-century life inventory.

For some, the gulf between their childhood dreams and their current reality seems so huge that they give up. They decide that this is it for them, and they spiral into regret and resignation. Others spin off in different directions. They suddenly start dressing like they're teenagers again. They take stupid chances with their careers, finances, and personal lives. They lose themselves in addictions to everything from booze to porn.

Perhaps worst of all, the middle years are also the time when our health is at risk. Doctors tell us that from here on out, we can expect our waistlines to grow, our muscles to shrink, our testosterone levels to plummet. A few short years ago we were invulnerable; now we're overwhelmed by pharmaceutical companies looking to take advantage of our flagging egos, reduced sex drive, loss of hair, and worries about our manhood. Pick your middle-aged neurosis and there's a pill for it.

All things considered, this whole middle-aged trip can seem pretty bleak.

I've come to believe, however, that the "midlife crisis" is not a crisis in the traditional sense of the word but rather a massive opportunity to claim or reclaim a sense of meaning in our lives. To grab hold of something resonant, significant, and substantial. When I see fellow forty-year-olds spinning out, I know it's really them saying—screaming—*I'm still alive!*

And that's actually a good thing. It's one of the major themes of *Your New Prime*: we *are* still alive. And the good stuff is just beginning.

We have to learn to embrace this phase in our lives not as a *crisis* but as an *opportunity* to thrive and live with vigor. At forty, we're probably less worried about money than we used to be: Men over forty have the greatest spending power of any demographic, accounting for over 40 percent of total consumer spending in the United States. We start more businesses now than we have in any previous time in history. Eighty percent of all money in savings accounts belongs to us. As a group, we New Primers have it pretty good!

More important than money, though, is the priceless gift of self-knowledge. We may not have all the strength or speed we had when we were younger, but by now we know ourselves— our strengths, weaknesses, hopes, and fears—far better than we did back in our twenties and thirties (when we acted like we knew everything). We know that focus and commitment are our friends, particularly when we want to make changes in our lives. We know that this whole "death" thing, whenever it comes knocking, isn't something we'll be able to talk, or buy, or cajole our way out of. It's coming. Maybe not now, maybe not in ten years, or twenty or thirty. But it's on the way, and if we don't squeeze every bit of passion, adventure, and joy out of these years that we can, we risk shuffling off this mortal coil with a raging case of the shoulda-coulda-wouldas.

This arsenal of hard-won self-knowledge, wisdom, life experience, and savings means that our middle years have the potential to be our best years yet—*if* we are prepared to commit to a better life.

That dedication begins and ends with making an ironclad commitment to great health. Taking immaculate care of ourselves—inside and out, from the heart, muscles, and plumbing to the brain, balls, and emotions—hasn't always been our strong suit. But now that we're coming up on halftime in this shooting match, we've got to make it a priority—especially if we want to live a full and vigorous life as we move forward.

We're in the driver's seat now more than ever with respect to our health. Though a few of the health problems we encounter as we age can strike unpredictably, the vast majority are what the fitness revolutionary Frank Forencich calls "diseases of affluence": Heart disease. Diabetes. Obesity. Depression. Erectile dysfunction. Low testosterone. Loss of memory and cognition. Loss of muscle mass and bone density. Cancer of the prostate and colon. Joint pain. Inflammation-related disorders. These are real problems, to be sure, but make no mistake: we bring them on ourselves through our sedentary, overfed lifestyles—particularly as we age.

The silver lining in this unbelievable irony is that *we can do something about it.* We have the power to banish or avoid nearly every health problem that regularly afflicts us. Getting everything tuned up, trimmed down, and running smoothly is the key to making the middle years your best yet. Even if you've never exercised, it's still in your power to turn things around: a 2009 study published in the *British Medical Journal* found that men who took up exercise in later life had health outcomes that nearly equaled those of men who had exercised consistently since their youth.

Vibrant health is the deciding factor in how this next chapter of your life goes. It maximizes your chances of living expansively, adventurously, and passionately for many more years to come. With it, you'll stay mentally and physically sharp enough to compete athletically and professionally in whatever arena you choose. Your confidence will soar, as will your sexual health and masculinity. You'll be willing to take the kinds of risks that will get you to the next level in your career and keep your marriage and family life thriving—all with the support of your newfound health and energy. You'll probably save money, too. After all, guys who take care of themselves spend way less on health care than guys who don't.

When I turned fifty in May 2013, I was one of the luckiest guys I knew. Professionally, I was doing what I wanted to be doing. I had three new businesses that I was excited to manage and run. My family was thriving. Physically, I was fitter than ever: I had just finished a single-day "Rim 2 Rim" run across the floor of the Grand Canyon. Two months later, I would complete the New York City Marathon. I was surfing the Maldives, skiing as much powder as I could find, climbing the Grand Tetons, and training regularly with some of the most accomplished athletes in the world—from UFC world champions to NHL players to the legendary surfer Laird Hamilton, who, at fifty-one, remains one of the fittest men on the planet. Through a commitment to a specific nutrition, lifestyle, and exercise regimen, I'd raised my natural testosterone levels by 36 percent in five years. When my AARP card arrived in the mail, I laughed and shredded it. For me, the idea of retiring right when things were getting good seemed patently absurd. Since then, I've built on those successes, and I continue to live a life I find incredibly rewarding.

In no small part, the life I have now, just a couple of years past my half-century mark, is the result of decades of research into the best ways to achieve and maintain peak health—physical, mental, emotional, sexual—through all stages of life. Twenty years ago, I embarked on this journey in order to stave off a number of serious medical problems that doctors told me were my genetic destiny—including prostate cancer and diabetes. Now I'm making it my mission in life to share what I've learned with you so that you can beat the odds as I did—and make forty and beyond *your* New Prime as well.

I've worn many hats over the years: Husband. Chef. Father. Lawyer. Developer. Cofounder of Boost Mobile USA. Private equity investor and venture capitalist. Health publisher. President of CooperativeHealth, PR Labs, and the Prostate Cancer Institute. More than anything else, though, health, fitness, and all aspects of peak performance—mine and yours—are my life's passion.

As you read *Your New Prime*, think of me as your personal channel to the best minds and experts in the field of health and wellness. Having spent all these years obsessively educating and surrounding myself with the best doctors, fitness experts, naturopaths, and nutritionists, and listening to and researching the real problems men face at our age, I know the questions that you want answered but are often too embarrassed to ask—particularly of a rushed and distracted physician who's giving you an average of fourteen-and-a-half minutes of his or her time.

Along the way, we'll focus on the things that matter. You won't need to train like a Spartan warrior. I couldn't care less if you achieve six-pack abs and seventeen-inch arms in three weeks, or twenty, or a hundred. Instead of giving you lots of muscle-building pep talks, I'll show you how to move well and achieve age-appropriate *functional* fitness that you can maintain and build on for the rest of your life. I'll tell you what to eat—and what to avoid—to feel and perform your best at every level. And I'll share techniques that will help you banish stress, ramp up your sex life, and top off your testosterone—naturally—so you can be your best in the bedroom, the weight room, and the boardroom, now and for decades to come.

Best of all, I'm going to chart out exactly how you can accomplish all of this in point-by-point instructions at the end of each chapter. These are instructions that you can (and should!) implement immediately—and then adhere to for thirty days. Follow these guidelines for thirty days, and you will see and feel changes in all areas, and you will set your life on a new and exciting path forward. Along with many changes in how you feel and look, you will also find a new purpose and vitality, and a direction that you may have worried you'd lost forever. The New Prime version of you will be closer to the man you always thought you could be, and the man you hoped you would become.

We're at a fork in the road, gentlemen. Down one path lies poor health, disillusionment, and a revolving-door relationship with hospitals and the health care industry. Down the other lies the richest, most rewarding years of your life.

I know the path I'm on, and the one I'm going to continue to take for the *next* half century. Care to join me?

MY STORY: EPIGENETIC FREAK

August 1980, the Gold Coast of Australia. I'm lying on an examination table, and my heart feels like it's trying to gnaw its way out of my chest. I can't move and I can't breathe.

I'm pretty familiar with the patterns of my cardiovascular system. At just seventeen, I have a résumé that reflects my compulsive hunger for sports of every kind: pro skateboarder, national-level surfing competitor, age-representative rugby player, state Tae Kwon Do champ. Before leaving New Zealand at age fifteen, I had also had my share of scrapes involving street gangs and other questionable types. I know a fast heartbeat.

This, however, is something completely new. Something is wrong.

Just half an hour before, I'd hung up my apron after the lunch shift at the restaurant where I work as a chef, wondering if I'd have time to catch some waves before sundown. But as I began the short trek back to my tiny apartment, I felt a vise-grip close around my heart.

Dazed, I'd stumbled into a naturopath's office, where a pair of therapists had begun trying to fix me with acupressure and herbs. All respect to people in their profession—I've since had good luck with many types of alternative therapy—but in this case, their efforts appeared to have been for naught.

His heart stopped! I hear one of them say, and for an excruciating fifteen seconds, the room turns into a flurry of activity as the familiar, reassuring *ba-boom, ba-boom* in the center of my chest falls silent.

That's an odd feeling, to say the least.

When it starts again—mercifully—I mutter something about feeling better, and I lurch out of the office to resume my zombielike shamble homeward (seventeen-year-olds aren't known for their good judgment). Maybe, I think, I'll lie down and feel better. Or failing that, I'll call an ambulance.

Just shy of the apartment complex, however, I collapse in a grassy field, unable to walk or move. As the blazing, 100-degree Australian sun makes spots across my vision, I wonder if this is what it feels like to die.

When I awake, I'm told that I was found in that field (by a nurse, as good fortune would have it) and rushed into surgery. I have an eight-inch vertical scar in the center of my chest, flanked by two smaller horizontal ones where a heart surgeon tapped me like a keg of stout and drained the better part of a liter of fluid out of my chest.

The condition that caused the pain, and might very well have killed me, is called pericarditis: a viral inflammation of the saclike membrane that surrounds the heart. The swelling can put pressure on the heart; it is often described using words like *mild*, *transient*, and *uncomfortable*—none of which remotely described my condition. In my case, the sac swelled so much that my heart literally couldn't pump.

Following the surgery, the surgeon tells me, almost offhandedly, "It very well might recur, and there's no way of knowing when it will, or what will bring it on."

Those aren't words you *ever* want to hear about a life-threatening condition. And when you're a seventeen-year-old surfer with a healthy disdain for mortality, those are words you can barely understand or process.

On the way home from the hospital, in the pouring Australian rain, my girlfriend (now wife of twenty-seven years) Maria pulls over in our $500 clunker, and we hold each other and cry like a pair of schoolkids over our uncertain future.

WAKE-UP CALL

Though I wasn't yet twenty, this was hardly the first high-level health scare I'd faced. As a teenager, I broke so many bones that the emergency room practically had a punch card for me (it was later discovered that I had osteopenia—or low bone density—which make bones more apt to break). At age nine, I developed encephalitis, or brain swelling, after a case of the mumps, and I was in a semicomatose state for a month under the care of a private nurse.

One Sunday two years after that, I crashed my dirt bike and sliced open my left shin on the chain. No emergency room was open, so a doctor neighbor of ours rinsed the wound with a garden hose, sewed me up, and sent me home. A charitable enough act, I suppose, but his failure to properly disinfect the wound landed me in the hospital again, this time with a bone marrow infection called osteomyelitis that threatened to eat through my entire leg. For five weeks, I lay in a hospital bed with doctors monitoring my condition, amputation saw at the ready.

Still: compared with being told I had an unpredictable, life-threatening heart condition, these other health crises seemed minor.

In retrospect, I realize that those heart-stopping fifteen seconds were a major transition point for me. My martial arts teacher refused to let me train at his studio. The coach of my rugby squad kicked me off as well. Even though my condition was not exercise-related, neither coach wanted to risk my dying on his watch.

Worse, my seventeen-year-old body—which had seemed so unstoppable on a surfboard, skateboard, or rugby field—suddenly appeared to be turning on me—not because I was overdoing it or getting injured, but because of bad luck and, it seemed, lousy genes. Though I looked strong and healthy, played hard, and felt great, my predisposition to viral inflammatory disease—which I believed back then was out of my control—was working against me.

From that point on, I resolved to take my health into my own hands as much as I could. My body had challenges and limitations, to be sure, but I was determined to beat them back with a fanatical commitment to health and fitness. I would maximize my chances of sticking around as long as possible, and live with as much energy, passion, and commitment as I could. If the medical industry offered me nothing but uncertainty, I'd do my own research and find my own solutions. Regardless of the lousy genetic hand I'd been dealt, none of my health challenges were going to sideline me. I was going to do everything I could to sideline *them*.

Collapsing in the middle of that grassy field was the first event that set me on the path I'm on now.

INTO THE MAD WORLD

A few years later, at the prompting of some professional types whose social circles I had stumbled into while playing on the local tennis circuit, I said an abrupt good-bye to my vagabond surfer lifestyle and showed up, uninvited and unadmitted, at the University of Sydney. Upon being told, by a very patient secretary, that I needed a little something called a high school diploma to be admitted, I enrolled in a community college. After studying sixteen hours a day and cramming two years of schooling into one, I graduated second in my class. It was good enough to actually get me into the University of Sydney that time. I took a double major in economics and law, graduating with honors, and briefly pursued investment banking and law before venturing out on my own as an entrepreneur.

A funny thing happened on my way up the corporate and tech-investment ladder. Increasingly, I noticed that the people I was working with were disconnected from both their bodies and from nature. While I took any chance I could to hit the beach for some surfing, take a trail run, go for a mountain bike ride, pump iron, or at the very least take a *walk*, my colleagues would sit at computers all day and then go home and watch TV or play computer games. On weekends they'd engage in more placid activities like concerts, golf, or movies. Success was measured not by how happy or fulfilled you were, not by the quality of your relationships or the passion with which you lived your life, but by how fast you made partner at the law firm or how big your annual bonus was. I actually remember one partner at the law firm where I worked who proudly trumpeted the fact that she was billing clients at the same time she was giving birth.

It made no sense to me: here were some of the most successful people in their field, and the concept of living a life of health and wellness was completely alien to them—it just wasn't a priority. Their diets were awful: convenience eating during the week, and rich, high-carb, calorically dense foods on the weekends. Stress was rampant in that environment, too, and before long, the people I knew—people with their whole lives ahead of them—were looking worse and getting more depressed. Some contracted diabetes, heart disease, or cancer. Other men were moving down a fast road toward those "age related" diseases that threaten to sap us of our masculinity—low testosterone, prostate problems, and declining energy and sex drive. The harder they worked and the higher they climbed, the sicker they got. Without the mixed blessing of a health-and-fitness wake-up call earlier in their lives, they had skated by on good genes and youthful vigor for many years, but now they were paying the piper in middle age.

I don't regret my time in the tech trenches. I still have many ties to that world, and I will probably always do business in it. But witnessing firsthand the toll that a highly competitive, stressful corporate lifestyle took on the health and fitness of many men my age was the second event that pushed me toward my new life as a full-time advocate for men's health and fitness.

ONWARD AND UPWARD

Genetically speaking, many of my buddies in the tech and business worlds were far more blessed than I was. But by any measure that mattered, I was far fitter and healthier: I was leaner, stronger, more positive, more energetic, and (if you want to get technical) I had better blood lipids and a better hormonal profile. Yes, my genetics were subpar, but—to invoke a new buzzword in the wellness lexicon—my *epi*-genetics were stellar. *Epigenetics* describes the aspects of one's genetic makeup that are profoundly affected by environment, diet, exercise, social interactions, family life, and other health-and-wellness-related behaviors. I had come to resemble Ethan Hawke's genetically inferior but fanatically focused character in *Gattaca*: innately disadvantaged, behaviorally exceptional. By maximizing the positive influences I could control, I minimized the effect of what I couldn't, and in so doing became what I jokingly refer to as an "epigenetic freak"—which so far is working above anyone's expectations.

At the time, I was just following my instincts—eating, exercising, and living my life in a way that seemed to maximize my health and fitness levels while minimizing my genetic liabilities. But in so doing, I had inadvertently stumbled onto a concept that's only just now gaining traction among medical experts. In his terrific book *The Disease Delusion*, Dr. Jeffrey S. Bland, widely considered the father of functional medicine, writes:

> The revolution that is changing health care is the recognition that our genes do not hard-wire us for chronic disease but instead offer us a menu of what we can be under differing environmental conditions. This is empowering. It means that at any age, we have a choice about what information we send to our genes from our environment, diet, and lifestyle.

This is a powerful message: genes aren't destiny, they're a menu of choices. And we place our order from that menu by how we eat, move, manage inflammation, interact with others, even *think*. We have to select carefully, though: the easy choices, like fast food and sedentary living and health-sapping chemicals that fast-track us toward chronic disease, are tempting, convenient, cheap, and pleasant—the "blue plate special" items on that vast menu. In *Your New Prime*, I want to inspire you to make better choices, and even a few off-the-beaten-path choices you may have to special order, that will put you on the road to vibrant health.

Now, I have plenty of respect for the medical profession. Some of my best friends are doctors. But I agree wholeheartedly with the belief that the health care industry, while skilled at treating acute problems, does very little for promoting long-term health, wellness, and disease prevention.

A few years back, I had a personal experience that drove this home for me. When I was forty years old, a routine blood test showed that I had abnormally high levels of prostate-specific antigen, or PSA. As a married, very active forty-year-old, I could barely allow myself to contemplate what that might mean: prostate cancer, incontinence, erectile dysfunction, and a sexless, impotent future.

My doctor's first course of action was a prostate biopsy—a procedure that is several orders of magnitude more unpleasant than it sounds—which showed no prostate cancer but an abundance of high-grade PIN, a precursor of the disease. At this point, my urologist informed me, the protocol was to repeat the biopsy every six months until they found cancer and then fast-track me into surgery, radiation, and the other treatments the medical industry depends on to keep its offices comfortably in the black.

Some people really do need the treatments they were offering me. What struck me about their approach, however, was that their only strategy was to wait around for cancer to rear its ugly head. Cancer, after all, is a clear, defined enemy, and doctors have tools to fight it for which they can bill patients and insurance companies extravagantly. By contrast, the medical industry knows next to nothing about preventative wellness—lifestyle and dietary adjustments you can make that might stave off cancer and other chronic illnesses for good. As someone who was cancer-free but at a high risk for contracting the disease, I desperately needed that kind of "treatment," but no doctor seemed able or willing to offer it to me. No one said, "Hey Craig, drink more green tea, eat more veggies, take a few supplements, and you'll probably have a better outcome." Nope. They just said, "Come back in a few months and we'll see if you're a candidate for next-level treatment." I was treated as a passive and potentially lucrative income stream.

Six months later I was lucky enough to meet Stuart "Skip" Holden, the medical director of the Prostate Cancer Foundation, who approached my case quite differently. Skip understood prevention. He understood my need to be fully informed and remain in charge of my own health. And under his guidance, I've stopped having biopsies. My PSA levels have continued to drop, and I'm healthier and stronger than ever.

If I'd chosen to live a different way—less disciplined, less positive, less scrupulous about the things I ate or the people I interacted with—I could very well be seriously ill or even dead right now. Instead, I chose to control the controllable in my life, and I'm thriving for it.

Here's a quick rundown of the health-and-fitness turnaround I've made, all of which was done using the techniques outlined in this book:

PROSTATE HEALTH

2004: PSA levels (the blood marker for prostate cancer) "high," cancer risk 30 percent.
2014: PSA levels "below normal," cancer risk *reversed*.

METABOLIC HEALTH

2004: Blood sugar over 100 ng/dL. Diagnosed as "prediabetic."
2014: Blood sugar consistently below 100 ng/dL. Diabetes risk *reversed*.

BONE HEALTH

2004: Osteopenia (bone loss) in evidence, high risk for osteoporosis.
2014: Bone loss reversed.

HORMONAL HEALTH

2004: Testosterone in midrange for a man my age.
2014: Testosterone 20 percent above upper range for most *twenty-year-olds* (816 ng/dL) and up 36 percent in five years—*naturally*.

BODY COMPOSITION

2004: Slow creep of body fat and loss of muscle mass.
2014: Body fat at 10.3 percent; increased muscle mass.

These are the kinds of measurable, life-changing results that are possible—in your forties and fifties!—using the methods in *Your New Prime*. They're the results I want for you, and for every other guy who's teetering on the brink of lifestyle-related diseases that have the potential to wreck his physical, mental, and sexual health. It's not too late to make a change.

Take an hour or two to skim through any well-regarded nutrition manual (such as Dr. John Berardi's *Precision Nutrition*) and you'll know far more about nutrition than the average American doctor knows about the subject upon graduation from medical school. Harvard Medical School, for one, doesn't have a *single* course on nutrition—not one! (Leading one to wonder what happened to the old adage "Let food be thy medicine.") It makes no sense that the people who are meant to be on the front lines of disease treatment have no training in disease prevention. Just think about it: When was the last time your doctor asked you what you eat—or anything about your nutrition, for that matter? Part of my intention with *Your New Prime* is to fill the gap left by the medical industry—the gap between managing disease and creating exceptional health.

Remember, I'm traveling this road right along with you, continuously looking for the best ways to stay healthy and avoid the nasty and chronic conditions that threaten the quality of life I've worked so hard to achieve. This book is my attempt to spell out what I think are the best practices for self-care for men as we get older. As you'll see, the book is divided into chapters that are further grouped into bite-sized chunks covering the high points of your health and wellness: diet, exercise, stress, sexual health. Feel free to read *Your New Prime* in random chunks, cherry-picking the sections that are most relevant to your life and needs—but remember that the rubber really meets the road when you start putting the concepts into directed action, as I recommend in the thirty-day plans outlined at the end of each chapter. I have no doubt that as time goes by, some of the information in this book will be supplanted by better, clearer, or simpler ideas (that's the point of science, after all). But now that we've reached middle age, we don't have time to wait around for the perfect solution to all that ails us. As we say in the business world, a good plan today is better than a perfect plan tomorrow.

All told, the plan outlined in this book, for your first thirty days and beyond, is designed to put you on a path to developing health consciousness—a day-to-day, minute-to-minute awareness of how each action you take, from the food you put in your mouth to the thoughts you allow into your head, affects your mental and physical health. One of the foundational points I'd like to get across in this book is that virtually every action you take has some effect on your health, and when you have a good grasp of those effects, you can make choices that move the needle in the right direction. If you're a man over forty, this book contains the best blueprint available on how to make that happen.

PART I

TOPPING OFF YOUR T TANK

Optimizing Your Life Force

CHAPTER 1

Supercharge Your T—Naturally

For thousands of years, men in China believed they could build sexual stamina and willpower by eating tiger penises. For the ancient Greeks, it was sparrow brains and the flesh of the skink, a rare lizard. To this day, male Australian Mardudjara aborigines eat their own severed foreskins as part of a circumcision ritual, believing it will hasten their initiation into manhood and make them strong.

The idea that something we eat, drink, inject, soak up through our pores, or even slice off our own bodies and devour whole can turn us into paragons of masculinity has been around since the beginning of time—and it's an appealing one. After all, true manliness is elusive and hard to define. And some guys—the quarterback marching his team down the field, the construction worker building a house from the ground up, the CEO leading the corporation to record profits—can make it all look so easy. Wouldn't it be great if there were a pill, potion, or powder that could distill it all down and confer manliness upon us, once and for all?

As men with a few years under our belt, we probably should be less susceptible to the myth of manhood in a bottle. By now, most of us have had experiences when we've manned up under pressure and others when we haven't, so we know that manliness isn't an all-or-nothing, you-have-it-or-you-don't proposition. We've also seen enough paragons fall from grace over the years—like heroes from Greek tragedy—to know that a life of perfect masculine virtue is pretty near impossible to pull off. Manliness is a moving target—as much a function of being adaptable and open to the demands of the moment as it is a finite set of rules or behaviors.

Still, the age-old idea of a magic-pill solution is a tough one to shake. And the drug industry, for one, banks on our faith in this idea. Big-time.

This chapter is about testosterone—the beneficial, androgenic (man-making) hormone we all produce naturally. I'm going to take a look at what this hormone does for us and outline the proven ways you can raise your levels without drugs to achieve new heights of vitality and vigor. It's not masculinity in a bottle—such a thing doesn't exist any more than femininity in a bottle does. Testosterone won't turn a soft-spoken, reflective guy into a road-raging hulk or a barroom brawler. But when you can train your body to produce more of it naturally, testosterone does seem to make you more focused, more energetic, and more vital—essentially, you become a more distinct and brighter version of yourself.

In the next chapter, I'll talk about *supplemental* testosterone, the latest and greatest of the cures for all that ails the post-forty male, including where this drug came from and why and how it's gaining traction with us New Primers. I'll outline the dangers of taking it, and what it can—and definitely *can't*—do for you. Finally, I'll take you through what you need to know if you do decide to start taking supplemental T, and what safety precautions you should observe once you're on it.

I'll be as objective as I can here, but I may as well lay my cards on the table right up front: whereas elevating your T naturally is one of the best things you can do for your health and vitality, taking *supplemental* T is a big mistake for all but a few of us—a veritable deal with the devil. But I'm getting ahead of myself.

THE STORY OF T

Evolutionarily speaking, T has been around for quite some time. It can be found in CEOs, football players, and horny guys in bars, but T also shows up in mammals, birds, and reptiles—and even fish and insects, in a slightly modified form. T has been with us since we crawled out of the primordial muck (and it may have even been a cause for crawling out of that muck, as high T is associated with risk-taking and rule-breaking).

As we all learned in sex-ed class, testosterone is the male sex hormone, responsible for all the stuff that happens to us in puberty—fertility, body hair, deep voice, big muscles, smelly armpits. In men, most of it is made in the testes, though a small percentage is made farther up, in the adrenal glands (in women, it's made in the ovaries, at 5 to 10 percent of the production rate of men). In addition to helping us mature, testosterone is also *anabolic*, enabling adult men to build and maintain muscle, strength, and bone density. Indirectly, it also appears to reduce the risk of cardiovascular disease by helping men reduce fat, lower cholesterol, and metabolize sugar more efficiently.

But when you're low in testosterone (a condition known as *hypogonadism*), your sex drive and sexual functioning drops. You may get fatter, lose muscle mass, and become depressed, listless, and unfocused. On the other hand, according to a Penn State study published in the *Journal of Behavioral Medicine*, a slightly above-average level of testosterone is associated with lower blood pressure, a healthy sex drive and sexual functioning, lower incidence of obesity, and an improved sense of well-being. Psychologically, it may also aid memory, attention, and spatial ability, and, according to a 2005 study from the journal *Neurology*, it may guard against the cognitive decline and dementia that affects many men as they age.

In general, higher T can also drive high performance. One interesting study, published in the *British Journal of Oral and Maxillofacial Surgery* in 2011, found that doctors' testosterone levels leaped up to 500 percent when they performed complex surgeries; the more complex the procedure, the higher the surgeons' T rose. But on an interesting side note, very high levels of T can also *impair* cognition (just think about road rage), indicating that there may be a "Goldilocks" level of T that's ideal for brain function. Plenty of research—and common knowledge—links high T with alpha-male, dominant, and sexually assertive behavior. T spikes in men who win athletic contests and plummets in men who lose; it also rises substantially following an encounter with a new sexual partner. New anthropological evidence suggests that a species-wide *drop* in T some fifty thousand years ago coincided with a sudden spike in cooperation, art, and technological innovation.

But recent studies have tempered the widespread belief that T turns us into knuckle-draggers. Many studies done on criminals find no clear association of higher T with violent behavior. Physical aggression and difficulty in school are actually associated with *low* T (and higher estrogen) in young boys, and social success and fair behavior—in both boys and adults—are associated with *higher* T.

In a word, if you could bottle what makes a man biologically "manly," for good and ill, testosterone is it. As Andrew Sullivan wrote in the *New York Times Magazine* in 2000, "Men and women differ biologically mainly because men produce 10 to 20 times as much testosterone as most women, and this chemical, no one seriously disputes, profoundly affects physique, behavior, mood and self understanding."

So though T sometimes gets a bad rap, in many ways it's great stuff—the stuff that makes life as a man at any age such a fascinating challenge. I'm not knocking art, creativity, cooperation, and a nurturing family life. Without those things, we'd still be bashing each other on the heads at every turn. But it's a balance. And though I'll stop short of saying that T is the solution to all that ails us as over-forty men, it is unquestionably a biomarker of the vitality and vigor we need to keep pursuing our dreams and pushing for the next frontier. In many ways, T is the stuff of Your New Prime.

THE MYSTERY OF DECLINING T

At present, our testosterone levels are under siege. Various factors appear to be pulling our T levels into the gutter—from sedentary jobs to poor diets and lifestyle choices to more ominous influences like environmental toxins. One particularly disturbing study, published in the *Journal of Clinical Endocrinology and Metabolism* in 2007, indicated that men's testosterone levels plummeted 17 percent from 1987 to 2004—and that's controlling for health and lifestyle factors, such as obesity and diabetes, that are known to affect T levels. The study found not only that individual men were losing testosterone as they aged (which is fairly normal), but that same-age men from later eras had substantially lower T than their predecessors: a man who turned 65 in 2002, for example, had much lower T than a man who turned 65 in 1987.

At the same time, males in the United States are experiencing an increased incidence of birth defects in the penis and testicles, a higher rate of testicular cancer, and a general decline in reproductive health.

Why are these things happening? The 2007 study suggests that although poor health in general is associated with a drop in testosterone, this generational decline cannot be fully explained by obesity, depression, or diabetes. Other studies—including one compelling study of 325 over-forty men by Dr. David Handelsman of the University of Sydney—have concluded that "age alone does not make you testosterone deficient." And natural selection couldn't solve the puzzle either; by all rights it would take generations to engineer such a massive shift in hormonal levels.

One possible explanation? *Transgenerational epigenetics*, a field that studies the ways in which environmental influences can be passed down from one generation to the next, just like our genetic coding. For example, animal studies have demonstrated that exposure to some toxic chemicals can result in epigenetic changes that can be inherited—thereby increasing the risk of chronic disease in the next generations.

So are unknown and noxious environmental influences robbing us of our T levels—and therefore our masculinity? It isn't clear—but it's possible.

Until we do know for sure, it's on us to do everything in our power to counteract the influences that *are* known to deprive us of our physical and sexual health. Many guys assume that the solution is to pump themselves full of the hormone through artificial means—a solution that, as I'll explain in the next chapter, isn't nearly as effective as many people believe, and that, for many reasons, I find highly problematic.

But T that *naturally* hovers on the higher end is generally a very good thing. Though some guys manage just fine with lower T, there's no denying that a naturally higher T level, which offers benefits like clear skin, low body fat, sound sleep, and good muscle tone, is a bellwether of overall health, and something that we older guys should strive to maximize. It's both a cause and an effect of good health, an indication that our virility and vitality are on an upward, rather than a downward, spiral.

Through careful control of my lifestyle habits—diet, sleep, exercise, stress relief—I managed to *raise* my T levels 36 percent, from 517 five years ago to 816 today—and I accomplished this during the same period—my late forties and early fifties—when most men find their levels plummeting. I did it naturally, and I've never felt better. So I can attest to the benefits of making positive lifestyle changes to give your T a natural boost.

Though the advice in this chapter is all scientifically valid, I'll also admit that my experience is anecdotal. I'm one guy—albeit a borderline obsessive one who has tracked the research and scientific trends around testosterone for decades now. But even if you follow the advice here to a T, you may not achieve exactly the same results I did. It's conceivable—though unlikely—that your actual T levels won't change that much.

My response to that: *It doesn't matter.* If you are contemplating going on hormone therapy because your T is low, or because of symptoms you are experiencing, I urge you, with every fiber of my being, to try the advice detailed throughout this book first. For the sake of your own health, make absolutely sure that the problems you are experiencing are due to your physiology rather than your lifestyle. Be sure, because otherwise, changing your lifestyle will help you feel better. Your sex drive will return. You will be more vital, more confident, more focused, more able to carry out whatever aspirations you have for yourself in this incredibly rich period in your life. And at the same time, in all likelihood, your T will also go up—but even if it doesn't, you will banish many if not all of the symptoms that are driving you to contemplate T therapy in the first place. And that matters far more than some number on a blood panel report.

Let's get started.

THE T AUDIT

In the last three to seven years:

1. Has a physician diagnosed you with low testosterone?

2. Has your sex drive dropped?

3. Have your erections decreased in frequency and quality?

4. Have you lost noticeable amounts of strength or muscle mass?

5. Have you gained more than ten pounds?

6. Have you had difficulty maintaining a stable weight?

7. Has your energy dropped?

8. Have you found it necessary to shave less often?

9. Do you feel less engaged, committed, and excited by your career, family, or hobbies?

10. If you are trying to conceive, have you and your partner had a difficult time becoming pregnant, or have you been diagnosed with a low sperm count?

11. Do you feel less sharp and focused?

12. Has your mood gotten worse?

13. Have you contracted diabetes, obesity, high blood pressure, or high cholesterol?

14. Do you routinely sleep less than seven hours a night?

15. Do you often feel stressed, anxious, and overwhelmed?

16. Do you avoid exercise?

17. Do you consume soy products (tofu, soymilk, protein powders containing soy) more than once a week?

18. Do you drink out of plastic bottles containing BPA?

19. Do you consume foods containing environmental toxins such as inorganic meats?

20. Do you use self-care products that contain environmental toxins? (Look for unpronounceable chemical names, particularly in shampoo.)

21. Do you avoid social situations, particularly those involving meeting new people?

22. Do you eat a low-carb or low-fat diet?

Any "yes" answers to questions 1–13 indicate that your testosterone levels may be dropping or have dropped; "yes" answers to questions 14–22 suggest that you may be in danger of causing your T levels to decline.

THE NEW PRIMER'S GUIDE TO AMPING UP YOUR T

There are three sections here: "Stuff that Works," "Stuff that Kind of Works (But You Should Do Anyway)," and "Stuff That Doesn't Work." Don't get the lists confused: prioritize the "Stuff that Works" list, sprinkle in the "Stuff that Kind of Works" tips as much as you can, and stay away from the other stuff.

Helping you raise your T to a healthy level is one of my big priorities, so many of the tips here refer you to other chapters of this book, where you'll get more specific breakdowns on how to integrate these practices into your lifestyle.

Stuff That Works

Lean Out

Abdominal fat increases the conversion of testosterone (and androstenedione, a precursor of testosterone) into estradiol, a female hormone. In turn, as estrogen increases, so does the tendency to store abdominal fat. As your T drops further, you'll be even more likely to accumulate abdominal fat—and fat everywhere else as well.

All told, the fatter you get, the less T you have. So if you're a heavier guy and can't seem to rouse the energy to get out of bed, much less hit the gym after a day at work, it may not just be the additional heft that's weighing you down, but also your exponentially worsening hormonal profile.

I'm lucky in that I've never been overweight. So you may think it's easy for me to say "Slim down and you'll raise your T." But I know that losing weight can be very tough; there are genetic and environmental factors that can stack against you to make losing a noticeable gut feel like a lifetime struggle.

I'm here to tell you that if you make it a priority, you can do it. I'm not overweight, because I have made it a massive personal priority to stay lean—it's a fundamental part of my personal health and wellness program, for all the reasons outlined in this book. I'm not going to promise you abs of steel, but with the right approach to diet and exercise, you *can* slim down—significantly. And if you slim down, your T *will* increase, alongside all the other health benefits of weight loss you'll receive. One 2012 study from the Endocrine Society found that when a group of over-forty prediabetic men lost weight, the incidence of low T in the group went down 50 percent.

I'll also add that you actually don't have to lose a huge amount of weight to reverse the T-sapping trend. Another study found that obese men who lost seventeen pounds (which is a manageable amount if you're substantially overweight) saw their testosterone level increase by 15 percent. Even if you stop the cycle of packing on five pounds every year or so and merely *maintain* your current weight, you'll be taking very positive steps in the right direction.

For more on fitness—and saying good-bye to that T-sucking gut—see chapter 4.

Lower Stress

Stress gets a bad rap in the twenty-first century. In reality, it's as essential to our health as air or water. Just as your muscles and joints become weaker and smaller without a certain amount of impact and strain, we get restless, bored, and unfocused without a certain amount of stress in our lives. We're made to absorb and deal with stress. Why go to sporting events, or participate in a sport, or even go to a movie or watch a TV show except to experience a vicarious sense of tension and drama?

Too much chronic stress, however, *is* harmful. Long-term chronic stress places an enormous load on your adrenal glands, leaving you fatigued, irritable, depressed, and turned-off. The stress hormone cortisol, produced in the adrenals, can also deplete the body of dehydroepiandrosterone (DHEA), which is one of the major building blocks of testosterone. In short: higher cortisol, lower T.

It's been theorized that, evolutionarily speaking, lower T was useful in times of high stress because the behaviors associated with high T—things like aggression, mating, and competitiveness—were likely to get you killed when the heat was on (remember that the hyperaggressive soldier type *always* gets eaten in the first reel of a zombie flick, while the rational, more cautious hero survives). These days, it's no longer tribal warfare and woolly mammoths that stoke our anxieties, but deadlines, angry bosses, and mortgage payments. Physiologically, however, the result is the same: high stress, low T.

Common stress relievers like yoga, meditation, deep breathing, positive visualization, and connecting with friends and family should be essential parts of your life anyway—but the additional boost these activities give to your T is yet another reason to commit to doing them regularly. For more tips and strategies, take the stress audit in chapter 6 and follow the guidelines provided.

Engage in Fast, Brief Cardio

When most guys our age think about losing weight or getting fit, one word comes to mind: *jogging*. For many reasons (some of which I cover in chapter 4), I want you to erase that idea from your mind.

I'll grant you this: when it comes to your heart and lungs, jogging may be better than doing nothing. But given the other liabilities that come with jogging, it may not win by much. Consider that jogging is a repetitive activity, particularly when done on flat pavement or a treadmill, where the terrain is hopelessly unvaried. Over and over and over again, you absorb up to seven times your body weight with each stride. Because the range of motion in your hips, knees, and ankle joints is limited, you gradually lose mobility in those joints. Jog for long periods and regularly enough, and you actually *lose* fast-twitch muscle mass in the large muscle groups of your thighs and hips—and the strength and power those muscle fibers provide erodes.

Most significant, your testosterone levels drop substantially as your mileage increases (if you're prepping for a marathon, for example). One study from the *British Journal of Sports Medicine* found that, in middle-aged long-distance runners, "training was inversely proportionate to testosterone levels"—the longer the men ran, the lower their T.

Studies aside, I find that many long-distance runners appear unhealthy. With the exception of the genetically gifted gazelles you see in the Olympics, marathoners typically look exhausted and emaciated. Compare your average marathoner with your average lean, muscular sprinter, and there's no contest: sprinters just look better.

If you're going to run, run fast—and intermittently. One 2010 study published in the *International Journal of Sports Medicine* found that testosterone levels increased measurably in young men after they performed sprint intervals on a stationary bike lasting just *six seconds*. It doesn't take much.

The bottom line is that we have a limited amount of time, and we need to train hard and fast in the time that we have—and make it count. For more on PRIME Workouts—the New Primer's preferred method of cardiovascular exercise—see chapter 4.

Catch More Zs

One important tactic in stopping the spiral down into the T basement? More sleep. If burning the midnight oil, getting up at the crack of dawn, and toughing it out all day with Red Bull makes you feel manly, be advised that it won't do so for long: most of the T you burn off during the day is replenished during sleep—so the fewer Zs you catch, the less time your body has to replenish those stores. One University of Chicago study found that men who averaged five hours of sleep a night experienced a 10 to 15 percent drop in testosterone the following day.

Older guys may be especially susceptible to the T-draining effects of skimping on sleep. One study found that young male rats who were deprived of sleep experienced a decline in testosterone over five days—but for older rats, the drop was even steeper, and it took longer for their T to return to normal when they resumed a regular sleep schedule.

Your mom was right: seven to eight hours of sleep a night is optimal for all-around health. When we were kids, we could afford to skimp a little more, but no longer. Get all the sleep you can—at night or in catnaps during the day.

FREE VERSUS BOUND T: WHAT'S THE DIFFERENCE?

If you get your T levels tested, you'll probably get a slew of numbers: *total, bio-available,* and *free.* What do these numbers mean?

Hormones act like commuters on a train: they circulate through the bloodstream, where they are often linked to other substances, then they get off when they reach their target tissues (like muscle and bone) where they are to perform their particular function.

Most of the time, T hitches a ride on something called sex hormone-binding globulin (SHBG). Less frequently, it binds itself to another substance called albumin, and still less often, it bodysurfs through your system solo.

As you probably can guess, "total" T represents all the testosterone in your system in *any* state—bound to SHBG, bound to albumin, and all by its lonesome. "Free" T is the stuff that's on its own. "Bio-available" T is a measure of free testosterone combined with the T that's bound to albumin. Generally speaking, about 65 percent of the testosterone in the blood binds to SHBG, 30 to 40 percent binds with albumin, and about 2 percent is free.

Here's where it gets tricky (and relevant to a guy trying to boost his sex drive, energy, and muscle-building potential): only the bio-available T—the free T plus the albumin-bound stuff—really matters. That's because when T is bound to SHBG, it can't jump off and do its job on the target tissue: it's as if it's handcuffed to the commuter train.

The difference between "bio-available" T and "total" T is a bit like the difference between body fat percentage and total weight. You might weigh a healthy sounding 180 pounds, but if 33 percent of that is body fat, you're definitely less than healthy.

So another way to effectively increase your T is to unleash a greater percentage of it from the SHBG that keeps it corralled. And lucky for you, this book includes several methods of doing just that.

Clean Up Your Diet

Many foods have been shown to cause a substantial drop in T. A 2009 study, for example, found that ingesting a solution of pure glucose (sugar in its simplest form) could suppress T levels by up to 25 percent for up to two hours afterward. Other research indicates that *dioxins*—a chemical family found in herbicides used to treat animal feed—can not only lower T levels, but also cause damage to the male reproductive system in other ways as well.

The takeaway here is that keeping T topped off means staying away from too much simple sugar and too many quick-digesting carbohydrates like pasta, bread, and desserts, which quickly convert to glucose in the body—though *don't* eliminate carbs or lower them too steeply, either! (See "Eating Low-Carb" in the section on stuff that doesn't work.) If you're going to eat these things, you should at least eat them with other foods that take longer to break down, such as protein and veggies. Also, consider avoiding conventionally raised meat products, especially fatter cuts of meat (dioxins accumulate not in the lean tissue but in the fat of animals we eat), as well as nonorganic, high-fat dairy products.

Eat Your Veggies

Cruciferous veggies like broccoli, cauliflower, and cabbage contain the phytonutrient (plant-based nutrient) indole-3-carbinol (I3C), a precursor to another tough-to-spell phytonutrient called diindolylmethane (DIM). Both I3C and DIM, which you can also take in supplement form, as I'll discuss shortly, do clean-up detail on the harmful, T-sapping estrogens in your body, while also helping combat prostate cancer and benign prostatic hyperplasia (BPH, an enlarged prostate). Take in these treelike veggies daily if you can. In general, veggies also help control inflammation (kale, spinach, and blueberries are especially good for this), which helps you stay lean and gives your T another added boost.

Go Green(er)

Xenoestrogens—chemical compounds that can ramp up estrogen production and dampen T—are unfortunately pretty ubiquitous. Here's a partial list of where these nasty substances can show up (brace yourself):

- Inorganic meat products.

- Chemical-laden cleaning products (choose plant-based cleaners whenever possible and check the labels for chemicals).

- Any personal care products (shampoo, deodorant, lotions) that contain the following ingredients (all of which are estrogenic): DBP, DEP, DEHP, BzBP, DMP.

- Most products with "fragrances," such as cleaning products, air fresheners, and scented candles. (Those made with essential oils are typically safe.)

- Most plastic containers for food and water, which contain BPA—a substance that mimics estrogen in the body. Use glass or stainless steel containers instead.

- Anything that has been heated in a plastic container. (I don't use a microwave for this reason!)

- Plastic bags. Here in California, they're now banned in many stores, so we're becoming a state of cloth-bag carriers. If your local store is lagging behind, opt for paper.

- Receipts. Surprisingly, about 50 percent of receipts contain BPA! Choose the email receipt option whenever possible. And when they ask, "Do you want your receipt in the bag?" say yes. Anywhere but in your hand.

That's a hefty list. I certainly don't want you to hide out in your organically scrubbed apartment, Geiger-countering the mail for estrogenic substances. But be on the alert for these things and see if you can figure out ways to limit your consumption and handling of them. At the very least, grab on to the concept that T-sapping xenoestrogen substances are in items all around us, and that going organic and natural with as many of the products you buy as possible is for the best. Your T levels will thank you for it.

Socialize More

Unsurprisingly, T gets a healthy boost when you interact with attractive women. One study found that when heterosexual men had a five-minute conversation with an attractive woman, it caused T levels to jump 30 percent (conversing with other men caused a smaller jump of 13 percent). It should be noted that T levels saw a similar jump *whether or not* the women seemed interested in the men—evidence (as if any more were needed) that we're sometimes as clueless as our wives and girlfriends say we are.

Finally, having actual sex causes T to increase as well. One study found that men over sixty who engaged in frequent sexual activity had significantly higher T than those who didn't. Watching sexually arousing videos also increases T, as does masturbation. Ejaculation—contrary to common boxing-gym wisdom—does *not* cause testosterone levels to drop substantially, though, through the action of a number of other hormones, it does tend to mellow you out for a time. T is a social hormone, so get out there and interact.

STAY AWAY FROM PHTHALATES

Earlier we talked about BPA, a chemical found in plastics that poses a big threat to your hormones and therefore your masculinity. Recently, information has surfaced about another group of chemicals—also found in plastics and personal health care products, among other places—that may be even worse.

"Phthalates" are even more of an insult to your system than they are to my spell-checker. They belong to the same class of pollutants as BPA, called "endocrine disrupting chemicals" (EDCs). And although phthalates have been studied extensively (and declared "safe," predictably, by interested parties), the true extent of the dangers they present is only now coming to light.

According to a 2014 study published in the *Journal of Clinical Endocrinology and Metabolism*, "exposure to phthalates, chemicals found in plastics and personal care products, is associated with reduced androgen levels and associated disorders." The study found that the presence of high levels of these chemicals in the urine of test subjects was associated with significantly reduced T levels in all the populations tested—men and women, young and old. There was a particularly pronounced reduction in boys ages six to twelve and men ages forty to sixty, for whom exposure was linked to a 13 percent decrease in T levels.

No pollutants are good, of course—but for men hoping to hang on to their masculinity hormones, phthalates are particularly nasty: the highest levels of phthalates are associated with all kinds of side effects from breast growth to infertility. So you're smart to keep these pollutants out of your home as much as possible, and away from your family as well. The trouble is, they're almost everywhere. Here's a quick list of a few places you're likely to find these chemicals:

- Plastic food and beverage containers, especially plastic-wrapped foods, such as meats and other produce.

- Hair spray and hair gel.

- Deodorant.

- Anything fragranced (soap, shampoo, air fresheners, laundry detergent, aftershave, face and hand lotions). If it's scented, you can bet it contains phthalates and other EDCs.

- Insect repellent.

- Cleaning products.

- Carpeting.

- New cars. That "new car smell" is nothing but the fine scent of phthalates.

- Vinyl flooring.

- Insulation on wires and cables.

- Shower curtains.

- Raincoats.

- Plastic toys.

- Steering wheels, dashboards, gearshifts.

- Medical devices (IV drip bags).

- Plastic sex toys.

- Sexual lubricants like K-Y Jelly.

- Cream-based dairy products.

- Pesticides found on conventionally raised fruits and vegetables.

Get the picture? Short of going off the grid, it's hard to imagine a life without some exposure to phthalates—which is probably why they are found in the urine of 95 percent of people tested.

So the key for New Primers is to get rid of as many of the highest-risk items as possible, using these few quick-and-dirty steps:

1. Go fragrance-free. Don't use anything on your body or in your home that has a fake-smelling odor. Clear out all scented cleaning and personal body products, and look for brands that are fragrance-free or that are made using natural plant-based oils—or that carry the Environmental Protection Agency's Design for the Environment seal. Use plain bar soap for shaving (see below) and coconut oil for moisturizing. Go all-natural for your shampoos and conditioners, and ditch the aftershave.

2. Store food only in metal or glass. Avoid any packaging with the 3, 6, and 7 recycling codes. Packaging with these codes may contain phthalates or BPA. Instead, look for recycling codes 1, 2, 4, and 5, especially for anything in which you carry, store, or cook food. Mason jars are great for leftovers. Use stainless steel containers like the Klean Kanteen for drinking water.

3. Microwave in glass. Forget "microwave safe": get some solid, high-quality glass or stainless steel containers for heating your food. Even supposedly "safe" plastics can leach EDCs into your foods at higher temperatures.

4. Go organic. Conventional agriculture is full of phthalates, thanks to pesticides—but not organic produce and meat. Get the good stuff whenever you can afford it. And avoid all meats that are wrapped in plastic—especially chicken—which often sit for days on display fermenting in E. coli bacteria. Buy the fresh cuts and get them wrapped in BPA-free paper. Wash all fruits and vegetables thoroughly.

5. Use nonsynthetic bar soap. Antibacterial soaps and body washes often contain triclocarban, another EDC that has been associated with testosterone disruption and prostate enlargement. Use a good old-fashioned nonscented bar soap. You get the same cleanup without the side effects.

6. Go filtered. Filter your water. It may not be perfect—some EDCs may still get through despite the filtering—but it's at least an ounce of prevention against some of the phthalates that show up in public drinking water.

7. Say N-O to the K-Y. Processed sexual lubricants contain chemicals linked to infertility, decreased sperm levels, and other endocrine-related disorders—not the stuff you want to be thinking about during sex. As an alternative, use coconut oil—it's antibacterial and a great lubricant, and it tastes a lot better than K-Y. It's also a great source of saturated fats that you can ingest in ways limited only by your imagination!

Supplement . . . Wisely

Flip to the back of just about any magazine whose readership is largely male, and you'll see a host of products promising to make you ooze T from your pores. Many are dispensable, and a few are a complete waste of money, but I believe some have enough legitimate science behind them to warrant your attention. Here are the best ones, which I take myself—and, full disclosure, I have also developed these into a formula for men that I highly recommend called EveryDay Male (see www.everydaymale.com for further details):

- **Vitamin D:** A deficiency of Vitamin D is associated with low T, so make sure you're getting enough. Vitamin D is found in fatty fish, cheese, eggs, and fortified products like milk, but this may be one vitamin that's best to take in supplement form, as it can be hard to get enough of it from whole foods.

- **Zinc:** Similarly, your T may drop if your zinc level falls below a certain threshold (though that doesn't mean that getting more zinc beyond that limit turns you into Superman). You can find zinc in lean meats, poultry, beans, eggs, nuts, and chickpeas. Supplement, if necessary, with 15 milligrams per day.

- **Avena sativa:** More commonly known as wild oats, Avena sativa inspired the expression "sow your wild oats." An extract from oats called avenacosides enhances the release of a luteinizing hormone, which in turn stimulates production of testosterone. Wild oats also boost sex drive and help support better erectile function.

- **Tribulus terrestris:** This is an herb that contains a saponin substance called protodioscin, which also seems to boost testosterone by stimulating the release of a luteinizing hormone. The herb also increases production of dehydroepiandrosterone (DHEA), which is a precursor of testosterone.

- **Green tea extracts:** Green tea extracts, including the catechins, can interfere with testosterone "glucuronidation" (a metabolic process leading to the breakdown of T), causing an increase in the level of circulating testosterone.

- **Stinging nettle:** This is an herb that has long been used to treat urinary tract problems, including those associated with prostate problems such as prostatitis and BPH. Stinging nettle also has an ability to interfere with the hormone SHBG, as noted by several researchers. It works by blocking the interaction between free testosterone and SHBG, thereby making higher levels of free testosterone available in the body.

- **Tongkat ali:** This is a tree that is native to countries in the Far East. In a 2012 study, seventy-six men with low testosterone were given 200 milligrams of tongkat ali daily for one month, after which over 90 percent of them had normal levels. In a more recent study, thirteen older, physically active men took 400 milligrams of tongkat ali extract daily for five weeks, after which the men showed a significant increase in both total and free T concentrations.

- **Magnesium:** A 2011 study of martial arts athletes and sedentary men indicated that a magnesium supplement of 10 milligrams per kilogram of body weight raised free and total testosterone levels both at rest and after exercise.

NEED A QUICK BOOST?

You've probably heard how body language is an essential component of how others see you. But it also has a profound effect on how you perceive *yourself*—and, not coincidentally, on your levels of the hormones associated with confidence, dominance, and stress. In recent years, Dr. Amy Cuddy has performed experiments in which she tracks the effects of various physical postures on key hormones. The results have been striking: just two minutes in a "power posture" results in an average 20 percent jump in testosterone and an average 25 percent drop in the stress hormone cortisol. Two minutes in a "repressed posture" had the opposite effect. In theory, a habitual sloucher who shifted into a power pose could boost his T by an astonishing 40 percent.

So what's a power pose?

In truth, power poses are somewhat predictable positions: reaching your arms overhead like a track star crossing the finish line; leaning back in a chair with your hands behind your head like a CEO taking a refreshing pause; standing with your hands on hips, chest out, superhero style. Repressed postures are various versions of collapsed, small, or curled-in poses (think of the position you probably assumed while hunched over a tiny desk, filling in answer bubbles on a standardized test).

In work settings, people in positions of authority tend to gravitate toward "dominant" postures, while lower-status workers gravitate toward repressed ones. Instinctively, it seems, people take on the body language appropriate to their "station"—thus reinforcing the perceived social order.

Is it any wonder, then, that so many people feel powerless and stressed-out at work? Without meaning to, they're sending themselves a powerful message, day in and day out, that they *are* powerless and stressed-out—a message that is then reinforced by their hormonal profile.

Cuddy's encouraging findings suggest that it doesn't need to be this way. Instead, you can fake it till you make it. In those moments when you're feeling stressed and re-pressed, go ahead and superman it up by putting your hands on your hips and puffing out your chest for a minute or two—and you'll feel better. Worried you'll look foolish? Head to the break room, an outdoor spot, or even the bathroom and go for it. The boss might notice that newfound confidence and reward you accordingly. Your T levels certainly will.

According to Cuddy, these power postures amount to more than mere posturing. "When people feel more personally powerful, they become more present," Cuddy says in a summary of her work. "Better connected with their own thoughts and feel-ings, which helps them to better connect with the thoughts and feelings of others. Presence—characterized by enthusiasm, confidence, engagement, and the ability to connect with and even captivate an audience—boosts people's performance in a wide range of domains."

Sounds like exactly what we New Primers are after.

Stuff That Kind of Works (But You Should Do Anyway)

Lift, Hard and Heavy

Exercise, particularly lifting heavy weights, increases testosterone—at least briefly. Studies from as far back as 1988 indicate that testosterone does jump significantly in response to exercise, especially compound-joint movements like squats, dead lifts, chins, and presses performed with weights equaling or exceeding 85 percent of what you can lift once (mean-ing you probably won't be able to lift a weight that heavy more than five or six times). The time between sets should hover around thirty to sixty seconds, and the workout duration should remain at or around sixty minutes. Since T levels are typically highest in the morn-ing, working out in the afternoon *may* result in a greater boost in average testosterone levels throughout the day. (For more tips on how to create a workout that conforms to these pa-rameters, see chapter 4.)

All that said, although "lift weights to increase your T" has been an axiom among the überfit for decades, it's actually unclear whether the temporary jump in testosterone brought on by strength training can have a noticeable impact on your long-term T levels. Still, those transient spikes in T will bring up your *average* T levels over the course of any day that you lift weights, and that certainly can't hurt.

Either way, strength training should still be mandatory for all of us. Since the proven, indisputable benefits of exercise—for things like self-esteem, blood flow, and confidence—

mimic many of the benefits of increased T (without the need to take drugs), the direct effect on T almost doesn't matter. Lift heavy and often (and safely!), following the parameters discussed in this book, and you'll feel like a new man—T numbers be damned.

Take a Few Other Supplements

The benefits of the following supplements are not as well documented as the supplements from the previous section. But as there's some literature to support these supplements, I'll mention them here for completists:

- Fenugreek, or Greek hay, often used in cooking, boosts libido and "may assist to maintain normal healthy testosterone levels," as noted in a 2011 study. There was also a 2010 study that suggested fenugreek may aid in muscle-building and fat-burning; another study showed that it boosts free testosterone.

- Resveratrol is a phytonutrient, antioxidant, and anti-inflammatory found in red grapes, onions, and several other foods. In addition to helping fight prostate cancer, resveratrol also promotes heart health and has been shown to enhance levels of testosterone by 50 percent in mice. While we aren't the same as mice, this is another one to experiment with.

- Chasteberry and licorice are naturally occurring substances that you can take in supplement form. Both have shown some effectiveness in lowering estrogen, which can have many of the same effects as raising T.

- Boron is a dietary trace mineral found in a wide variety of foods such as almonds, avocados, broccoli, oranges, beans, bananas, red grapes, onions, and walnuts. Although the supplementation of this mineral is usually associated with treatment of menopausal symptoms and bone health, some research indicates that taking boron can raise levels of free testosterone as well. One study published in the *Journal of Trace Elements in Medicine and Biology* demonstrated that consuming 10 milligrams of boron with breakfast may cause a significant decline in SHBG, an increase in free testosterone levels, and a significant decline in estradiol.

- Ashwagandha, a woody shrub long used in an ayurvedic medicine to enhance mood, has showed some ability to boost serum testosterone in men after 90 days of use.

- I3C and DIM, two phytonutrients found in cruciferous vegetables, can also be taken in supplemental form, which may aid in restoring the balance between estrogen and testosterone in the body.

For the record, I take everything on this list—and I wouldn't recommend these supplements if I didn't.

FAST CAR . . . HIGH T?

Maybe there's something to that midlife sports car purchase after all. A 2009 study of young men monitored their testosterone responses to driving different types of cars for an hour: first, a decked-out Porsche 911 and then a sixteen-year old Toyota Camry. No shocker: the cruise in the Porsche caused a spike in T, while the ramble in the Camry caused it to flatline and sometimes plummet.

Researchers noted that while T stayed elevated throughout the hour in the car, the strongest T response came when drivers eased the Porsche through populated areas, where eligible females could potentially catch a glimpse of them. Such competitive display–type behavior—known as "peacocking" in the pickup world—often results in a surge in T.

Having owned a handful of thrill rides in my day (and having transitioned to a far more eco-friendly Prius in recent years), I'd wager that if those same guys had shelled out the $75K to own that Porsche, any boost to their T-levels in response to driving it would be negligible six months later—and might even be lower, due to the shock they would get whenever the monthly bill arrived. You want to be a peacock? Build a great physique—no monthly payments required.

Drink Coffee

Caffeine—and coffee in particular—appears to boost athletic performance and reduce inflammation, and it may give your T a boost as well. One small study, conducted on people who had undergone a two-week abstinence from coffee, found that after four weeks, men drinking caffeinated coffee increased their total testosterone and decreased their concentration of estradiol, whereas men drinking *decaffeinated* coffee did not. After eight weeks, however, the differences leveled off.

For self-experimenting types, that means you'll probably get the biggest boost out of caffeine by cycling it: abstaining for a couple of weeks, then going back to it when you need a little extra edge. I know one guy—a competitive runner—who drinks virtually no caffeine year-round, then loads up on it on race day. He swears by that technique, and if you're that disciplined, go for it. Other athletes I know use flat Coca-Cola on race day instead of traditional sports drinks. Personally, I drink a fat-enriched blended matcha tea smoothie with MCT oil prior to training, in order to activate fat-burning and power me through my workouts (for the recipe, see chapter 4).

Practically speaking, even if you cycle it, caffeine is never going to turn you from a muskrat to a musk ox. Still, a little joe won't hurt your T levels, either, and because of its other benefits (improved alertness, focus, and athletic performance, reduced inflammation), guys over forty may want to drink a cup or two a day. Just pass on the cream and sugar.

Take an Ice Bath

Submerging some or all of your body in ice water may not be the first thing, or the most pleasant thing, you think of when considering postworkout relaxation techniques. But it may be one of the best ways to promote recovery—and possibly get a T boost as well. After a workout, your blood vessels are dilated, and your muscles are filled with the byproducts of your labors, including soreness-inducing lactic acid. When you ice the affected area—or dunk yourself in ice water completely—your blood vessels constrict, effectively wringing those byproducts out of the muscles. When the icing ends, your blood vessels expand again, pulling freshly oxygenated blood back into the muscles and speeding the repair of the tissues.

During my group training sessions with Laird Hamilton, he has us alternate ice baths with time in a sauna, facilitating the return of oxygenated blood into the tissues. I also keep a commercial ice bath and an infrared sauna at home, which I've been using for the last five years—the same period in which I managed to boost my T so dramatically.

For most guys, installing an in-home ice bath is probably going a little overboard. But the DIY version is pretty easy: run the tub (cold water only) and top it off with three to four big bags of ice (or enough to make a solid two-inch-thick layer of ice in the tub). The first few times out, submerge your lower body only (I recommend wearing shorts to avoid any ice-to-skin contact on delicate areas) and stay in for five minutes at a stretch. Over time, work up to full-body immersion for ten to fifteen minutes at a stretch—or as long as you can handle it!

You will curse. You will question your judgment and possibly the existence of a merciful force in the universe. But when you get out, all will be forgiven, because you will feel amazing.

A less-hardcore option is to stay out of the tub and rub ice directly on the areas you trained: thighs, calves, chest, or arms. For this method, you can steal a tip from the athletic-training world and use ice-filled Dixie cups, peeling back the paper cup to expose more ice as it melts. This method allows you to massage an area at the same time as you ice it—another excellent recovery technique.

The burning question, however, is "Will it boost T?"—and the answer is "perhaps." One reason your balls hang outside your body (besides leaving them vulnerable to swift kicks) is because high temperatures limit sperm production. The following studies have also suggested a link between temperature and testicular functioning:

- A Japanese study found that, for DNA synthesis, sperm production, and "most likely" for testosterone production as well, the optimal temperature is 87 to 96 degrees Fahrenheit—a few degrees below body temp.

- One animal study found that exposing rats to high temperatures substantially lowered testicular weight and testosterone production; two others demonstrated that the Leydig cells of monkeys and rams secrete testosterone more effectively when cooled than when exposed to heat.

- In a 2013 study, researchers studying 6,455 men over a period of three years found that sperm quality, volume, and motility were significantly higher in the colder months of the year (making you more fertile during winter months). Since the same hormones stimulate sperm production and testosterone production, cold may help you crank out more T as well.

- I'll also add that colder temps in general may enable fat loss, lower inflammation, and, at night, facilitate better sleep, particularly in those of us who exercise a lot and whose core temperatures tend to run a little hot (pro athletes, for example, almost always prefer to sleep in a colder room). Better sleep, as I mentioned earlier, facilitates higher T. Most studies agree that a temperature above 60 and below 67 degrees Fahrenheit is optimal for sleeping, while temps below 54 and above 75 are disruptive.

Of course, none of these studies points to a clear connection between the *very* cold temps of an ice bath and optimal testicular functioning or T levels, and that's why I'm relegating ice baths to the "probably works" list. But it's not a bad idea to cool down your body—including your

---

WILL A SEX FAST BOOST MY T?

Going without sex may seem like a counterintuitive means to higher T. After all, what's the use of firing up your libido if you can't put it to good use? But a recent study has suggested that committing to a sex fast now and then may temporarily raise your T levels. Researchers measured the endocrine response to orgasm both before and after a three-week period of sexual abstinence, and found that after the break men had a higher spike in T levels postejaculation.

I realize that this idea may be impractical, and possibly stupid. I imagine it might be difficult to explain to a willing sexual partner that you "have to take a pass to-night" because you're trying to boost your T without coming across as a complete idiot, or risking a knee to the groin the next time you want some action. Still, it does suggest that the sex breaks that befall most of us from time to time aren't going to turn us into geldings, and that they may even have hormonal benefits. Just don't tell your partner.

---

balls—after exercising. And there's no question that cold therapy makes you feel great (after it's over!) and will definitely improve your recovery from your workouts. Unlike a lulling warm bath, it also wakes you right up.

Stuff That Doesn't Work

Long, Slow Aerobic Exercise

Long, slow aerobic exercise, like long-distance running and cycling, or long workouts of ninety minutes or more, can cause testosterone to flatline or drop. Some long-distance cyclists even have to get on T therapy simply to get their levels back up to something approaching normal. (Hours on a bike saddle, with all that weight where the sun don't shine, can also lead to erectile dysfunction—yet another reason to limit your long-distance exercise!) Low T in endurance athletes is a double whammy, because it can also lead to osteopenia and osteoporosis—low bone density—which makes these athletes more vulnerable to fractures forming during their sport of choice. I hate to knock any particular form of exercise, especially since so few of us get enough of it anyway. But if you're concerned about low T, stay away from all those junk miles.

Eating Low-Fat

There's a reason that injectable T is administered in an oily solution: it's fat-soluble. Cutting fat out of your diet—or even lowering it substantially—can reduce T levels. One study indicated that a diet consisting of less than 40 percent fat (with that fat coming mostly from animal sources) can lead to a decrease in testosterone levels. Another study showed that increasing fat consumption from 20 percent of total calories to 40 percent increased T levels significantly. Conversely, following a low-fat, high-fiber diet (ironically, the type of diet that was strongly recommended for optimal health even up to a decade ago), *reduces* testosterone by 12 percent. While 40 percent is an awfully high percentage of your diet to come from fat calories, this fact certainly drives home the point that dietary fat is important. So make (the right) fat your friend. More on this in chapter 3.

Eating Low-Carb

After the Great Dietary Fat Scare of the 1980s and 1990s turned out to be overblown, the Twenty-First-Century Carb Crackdown quickly took its place. Carbs stand accused of all manner of crimes, from expanding waistlines to brain fog to, invariably, diabetes and obesity.

When it comes to overly processed junk food (corn syrup–laden desserts, Wonder Bread, Saltines, sugary cereals), I couldn't agree more: that stuff's nutritionally bankrupt crap. But legitimate *whole-wheat* products, eaten in moderation, are another story entirely—the much-maligned bread and pasta included, which have caused all kinds of objections.

A recent study in the journal *Life Sciences* found that men who ate a high-carb diet for ten days had *higher* T and lower levels of cortisol (the stress hormone) than men who ate low-carb during the same period. If you exercise regularly (or perhaps plan to start exercising regularly soon), a low-carb diet is an even worse idea. In 2010, researchers studied the effect of low-carb dieting on athletic performance and found that after just three days of low-carb dieting, most subjects were unable to complete a cycling test. After three days back on carbs, they completed the test with ease.

Low-carb dieting, then, results in lower T, higher cortisol, and a drop in athletic performance. And since exercising hard and heavy is one of the most potent ways to up your T, eating low-carb is, effectively, another double whammy against your T levels.

I'll discuss this in more detail in chapter 3, but don't take this advice as a license to chow down on carbs of *any* kind: consumption of an exceptionally high-carb meal results in a temporary drop in circulating T. *Moderate* carb consumption seems to be the way to go.

THE INTERMITTENT FAST

I'll cop to it: I eat no solid food on Tuesdays. I'll have a sip of this or that here and there, and plenty of water, but nothing solid, and certainly no huge, gut-busting smoothies. It's a very ascetic day for me.

I do this for lots of reasons—weight control, body composition, and just-plain variety among them—but I also do it because it boosts my T. Intermittent fasting (IF) has been shown to increase your satiety hormones (the ones that make you feel full), including insulin, leptin, and adiponectin—which in turn boost T.

IF isn't for everyone. I'll admit, a day off from eating, even on a Tuesday, can disrupt your social life a bit. But it's something I've come to enjoy, and I know it does good things for me. During "hell week" in their training, Navy SEALs go almost a week without food (or sleep, for that matter), and emerge knowing that they can handle more—much more—deprivation than they thought they could. A weekly fast is a miniscule version of that same kind of self-imposed discipline. Give it a try at least once. You'll find that being hungry won't kill you—and without mealtimes to interrupt you, you'll probably have a very productive day, with a healthy T boost to go along with it. At the very least, you'll realize it's *not* impossible to function without gorging yourself every few hours. And that can be remarkably empowering.

Eating Soy

Stroll through the aisle of your average GNC or Vitamin Shoppe and you'll see tons of protein powders loaded up with soy. There's a reason: soybeans are cheap and plentiful, and it's easy to grind them up and make them into protein-filled powder (usually called *soy protein isolate* on the label) that consumers think will help them build muscle.

My advice is to stay away. After years of back-and-forth wrangling, researchers have demonstrated conclusively that if you're trying to hold on to your cojones, skip the soy. In active men, soy protein lowers T and raises cortisol—the stress hormone that most of us already have plenty of. Estrogen levels may also be affected, and not in a good way: one study (in which subjects admittedly ate soy in huge quantities) showed that some of the male subjects developed breast enlargement and nipple discharge. Yikes.

Read the labels on your protein powder, and skip the tofu at the local vegetarian joint.

Boozing It Up

Here's irony for you: many of the behaviors we associate with a certain type of over-the-top masculinity—staying up all night, wreaking havoc of various kinds, and, yes, boozing—are associated not with high T, but with *low* T. So the next time you meet an obnoxious, hard-drinking hell-raiser, just know he's probably compensating.

Plenty of studies confirm this, including a recent one that discusses the effect of alcohol on the hypothalamic-pituitary-gonadal (HPG) axis—the hormonal network that affects male reproduction. Turns out that alcohol not only lowers T but generally lowers fertility as well—a fact that may have been welcome news back when you were a tipsy teenager looking for action on a Friday night, but probably not so much now that you're an adult trying to hang on to your T.

Other reasons alcohol is tough on T: it promotes weight gain and causes damage to the liver. Packing on weight, as I discuss earlier, increases estrogen and lowers T, while overtaxing the liver—an organ also responsible for metabolizing T—can dampen your levels still further. That makes booze a double—or even a *triple*—whammy against healthy T levels.

I'm not going to preach total abstinence here—life is short and many of us enjoy a drink now and then. But I will say that the less alcohol you drink, the better off your T will be: studies have indicated that even two drinks a day can depress your levels. And drinking beer, specifically, is a huge mistake: hops, a key ingredient in the brewing process, are so effective at increasing estrogen that they are currently being studied as a way to treat hot flashes in menopausal women.

These are the by-the-book recommendations for guys who want to minimize the effect of booze on their T. Some guys enjoy beer or vodka sufficiently that they'll sacrifice a little T to get an occasional buzz. As with any health advice, there's a balance to be struck.

I probably don't need to add that drinking lots of alcohol is also a great way to pack on a gut, lose fitness and focus, and, if you go far enough with it, ruin your life. We've all known guys (and women, and young people) who have let the bottle steal vital years from their lives. If you have a problem with alcohol, get help for it.

WHAT ABOUT PROTEIN?

The caveman in all of us would probably like to believe that a high-protein diet boosts testosterone: you spend the day hunting the elk, you drink its blood and eat its flesh, it makes you strong and manly.

Sorry. Stuffing yourself morning to night with flesh of one kind or another (as some obsessive Atkins proponents do) won't up your T—and according to one small study from 2008, it might even lower it by boosting insulin-like growth factor (IGF), which interferes with T production. So as far as T goes, eating either way too much or way too little of any of the three major macronutrients (carb, fat, and protein) is wrongheaded.

Still, protein is essential for building muscle and repairing tissue, as well as for satiety. And protein also contains branched-chain amino acids, a potent muscle-builder and promoter of T levels. So though you probably shouldn't pound down an 84-ounce porterhouse every night, you should make sure you're getting enough good-quality protein throughout the day—from vegetarian sources, salmon and sardines, and some organic meats (more on this in chapter 3). And you shouldn't worry about getting too much.

YOUR THIRTY-DAY ACTION PLAN
FOR NATURALLY INCREASING TESTOSTERONE

Admittedly, that's a lot of information I just threw at you, and some of those tips by themselves require serious time and attention. For the sake of convenience, I'm going to distill things into concentrated ideas that you can put into practice right away as you get going on the first thirty days of Your New Prime. Of course, you'll get the best results from this chapter if you can put all these ideas into practice starting on day one. But I live in the real world too, and I know how difficult that might be. Instead, you can choose a handful of tips (buying organic vegetables, sleeping seven hours a night, and meditating once a day) to implement on day one, and then sprinkle in the rest as the month goes on, so that by day thirty, the whole plan is up and running. The key to this approach is to start with the changes that are easiest to make—those you are 90 to 100 percent sure you can adhere to—and then work up to the tougher ones. Better to get a few easy wins in early on before you tackle the tougher stuff.

Here are your main goals for naturally increasing your testosterone levels:

1. **Go hard and go home.** When exercising, focus on hard, fast cardio and strength training (for more on this, see my tips in chapter 4).

2. **Chill out.** Practice stress-management techniques and implement a once-a-day meditation practice as described in chapter 6.

3. **Hit your sleep target.** Aim for seven hours of sleep a night—no more, no less. For tips on sleep, see chapter 6.

4. **Eat organic** as much as you can afford to do so, and emphasize cruciferous vegetables like broccoli, cabbage, and cauliflower in your diet.

5. **Control your exposure to contaminants that raise estrogen and suppress T.** Audit your personal and household products (shampoo, soap, and so on) for any synthetic chemicals, especially those containing phthalates. Replace them with natural, nonfragranced products. Avoid touching or being exposed to any products with BPA, including plastics (especially those labeled with a 3, 6, or 7) and paper receipts.

6. **Handle and store food wisely.** Use the microwave as infrequently as possible, and use a glass container when you do. Switch your storage and drinking containers from plastic to glass.

7. **Socialize more.** Need more pals? See chapter 6.

8. **Skip the soy**, including products containing soy protein isolates (commonly found in protein supplements).

9. **Practice moderation.** Limit your alcohol intake to no more than one drink a day, experiment with fasting up to one day a week, and periodically abstain from ejaculation for a week.

10. **Supplement as needed.** Make sure you have enough Vitamin D and zinc in your diet, and supplement if necessary, experimenting with the natural supplements detailed in this chapter.

11. **Get cold.** Experiment with ice baths and with sleeping in a colder-than-normal room with fewer blankets.

12. Fake it and make it. Use body language and posture that conveys confidence and ease—both to others and to you.

13. Drink filtered water only, from stainless steel or glass containers.

Diet, exercise, sleep, stress management, socializing, supplementing. In many ways, this list summarizes the New Prime lifestyle, a lifestyle that will not only boost your T but also help extend and improve your life, give you energy, increase your libido, and give you a more positive outlook. Make good on these commandments 80 to 90 percent of the time and you'll be well on your way to achieving all of those things faster than you thought possible.

There's one more practice, of course, that I haven't covered here, one that has a *huge* influence on testosterone levels: the kind you get from a doctor and inject with a needle. And that's the subject of the next chapter.

CHAPTER 2

Skip the T Party

Why Supplemental Testosterone Is a Deal with the Devil

THE PRECURSOR: VIAGRA

It may be difficult for some of us to recall, but there was a time when talking about your member—much less admitting you had a *problem* with it—was a major taboo. Sure, locker rooms, bars, and other typical male haunts have always been home to big-fish stories about sexual conquests and the caliber of our equipment, but talking about your penis in mixed company just wasn't considered gentlemanly.

Then, like a tidal wave, Viagra crashed onto the scene.

The year was 1998, but you probably remember it like it was yesterday. While investigating the health benefits of a drug called Sildenafil, scientists at the drug company Pfizer found that while the drug didn't boost cardiovascular health as they'd hoped, it did have a huge effect on potency. The new drug, named Viagra (rhymes with *Niagra*, as in a huge, endless, gushing flow of insurmountable power), was marketed as a cure for erectile dysfunction (ED)—and an empire was born. In the first few weeks after it was released, close to forty thousand prescriptions for the drug were filled, and by 2008, sales reached nearly $2 billion.

It made no difference that Viagra was, and remains, a ready-made punch line (Jay Leno told 944 Viagra jokes between 1998 and 2002). By selling ED as a serious medical condition on the one hand, and hiring the former presidential candidate Bob Dole and the NASCAR star Mark Martin as tongue-in-cheek Viagra spokesmen on the other, Pfizer helped fuel one of the biggest blockbuster drug sales in pharma history.

At the same time, the company also discovered an untapped, highly lucrative market: Us. Aging men, looking for the twentieth-century equivalent of the skink lizard. Those millions of prescriptions were the first indication that guys of a certain age were not only willing but eager to reveal and discuss problems with sexual functioning, now that a simple and apparently harmless solution was available to them. Recreational use became common. Jokes or no jokes, the drug was a phenom.

The Viagra craze confirmed that if there's a drug out there that can make men our age feel better about insecurities relating to our manhood, we would be willing and ready to buy in.

Here's the funny thing: in the last few years, even as more of us are aging into Viagra's target demographic, the sales of the drug have flagged. Was it overhyped? In his 2003 book *The Viagra Myth: The Surprising Impact on Love and Relationships*, the urologist Abraham Morgentaler argued that Viagra works at a cost to the man taking it—and to his relationships with his sexual partners. It can't save a failing marriage. It can't restore a sense of identity or one's potency outside the bedroom. Indirectly, it may even lead to more insecurity: researchers in Australia found that Viagra commercials *created* sexual anxiety in men. Manhood, no surprise, is deeper and more complex than the ability to perform sexually over and over again at the drop of a little blue pill, and perhaps this decline in sales suggests that consumers have started to figure that out.

None of that matters to the drug manufacturers, of course: for now, they're continuing to pull in substantial profits from the pill, and to play blatantly on our insecurities at the same time. I recently met an actor who has made a small fortune from starring in ads for ED medications. At six-five, 240 pounds, with single-digit body fat, he's built like a linebacker. The only indication that he's over thirty-five is a slight salt-and-pepper in his hair. Subtle these advertisers are not.

Most disturbing to Pfizer is the fact that the patent for Viagra is due to expire in a few short years—2019, to be exact. Even with its sales down from the heyday of the first decade of the 2000s, that will mean a huge nosedive in profits for companies that make Sildenafil-based ED drugs.

As a result, big pharma has been scrambling to find the next Viagra—the newest, latest version of manhood in a pill. And they have found their answer in supplemental testosterone.

Supplemental testosterone is a drug that the FDA has officially approved only to treat hypogonadism, a serious medical condition in which a man's body, due to injury, chronic disease, genetic predisposition, or exposure to environmental toxins, produces little to no testosterone. But it is increasingly being prescribed off-label to treat far less serious and far more common conditions: low sex drive, weight gain, depression, low energy—a symptom list that conveniently bundles some of the more ubiquitous male health concerns under one name: "low T."

Prescription testosterone hasn't been tested or studied rigorously in the long term. It has many proven and very troubling side effects—and it may have others we don't know about yet. Perhaps most ironically of all, prescription T may be completely ineffective at solving the problems its manufacturers claim that it will.

Due to these disturbing initial findings, and to the increasing popularity of supplemental testosterone as a "lifestyle drug," the FDA is currently in the midst of reassessing safety.

But in the meantime, the industry is expected to swell to $3.8 billion in the next three years, almost double the value of Viagra at its high-water mark.

Welcome to testosterone replacement therapy. Let the buyer beware.

THE ALLURE OF T

Testosterone was discovered and isolated back in the 1920s and '30s—right around the time that our dads were born. Back in 1939, two scientists, who later won the Nobel Prize for their work, discovered that giving the drug to neutered chickens caused the birds to turn, physiologically, into roosters. Voila: instant chicken virility.

As far back as the 1940s, athletes, soldiers, and other professionals whose jobs required physical strength and stamina have been using T in one form or another to gain a competitive edge in their chosen activity. And the drugs delivered. From East German Olympic athletes right up through high-profile pros like Lance Armstrong, Ben Johnson, Alex Rodriguez, Barry Bonds, Floyd Landis, and Marion Jones, athlete after pro athlete has used steroids, often in the form of testosterone, for one simple reason: they work. (Steroids are synthetic drugs that mimic the naturally anabolic effects of testosterone.)

"Steroids are incredibly effective," says the Harvard-based steroid expert Dr. Harrison Pope in a recent documentary on performance-enhancing drugs. "A young guy who eats badly, sleeps badly, smokes, drinks too much alcohol, misses half of his gym workouts and takes steroids can blow away the most dedicated, most gifted athlete who does not take steroids in terms of building strength and muscle mass."

Steroids accomplish this by accelerating recovery from exercise. Strenuous exercise causes a breakdown in muscle tissue from which the body usually requires about forty-eight hours to recover (longer as we age). Like anabolic steroids, natural T accelerates and accentuates that recovery ability, allowing you to work out harder and bounce back more quickly from challenging workouts. It also hastens tissue regeneration system-wide, leading to faster recovery from injury and fewer of those aches and pains you may have decided were your lot in middle age. Result? A level of muscularity and leanness that's tough to achieve any other way.

Few of us are even serious amateur athletes, much less pros. And unless we're willing to turn to the black market, exercise like maniacs, and take levels of T up to ten thousand times the therapeutic dose (which some athletes do), we're not going to achieve those superhuman results. But athletes on the field of play nevertheless embody many of the qualities that New

Primers are striving to bring into our daily lives: strength, focus, determination, power, and a will to succeed and thrive under pressure. And as a group, they also tend to look healthier, more vibrant, and more alive than your typical cubicle-dweller. Plus, unlike pro athletes, we don't have to worry about drug tests. If so many of our highest performers rely on these drugs to reach the heights they've risen to, could supplemental T help nudge us a little closer to our own potential as well?

It works for chickens. It works for athletes. Most of us remember, dimly, that testosterone worked for *us*, too, back in our adolescence when we sprouted from pipsqueaks to hulks over the course of a few short years. It's natural and it seems to serve as a way to remain youthful and vigorous Peter Pans. What's not to love about this stuff?

HGH—THE OTHER MAGIC DRUG

Testosterone isn't the only prescription drug offered up as the fountain of youth by the burgeoning "antiaging" industry. At many "low T" clinics, human growth hormone, or HGH, is the foundation of the program, especially in image-conscious Southern California, where it is the drug of choice for celebrities and movie stars.

There's a reason for that. When your HGH is topped off, it promotes cellular repair, helps grow muscles and bones, and aids in the breakdown of subcutaneous fat. Like testosterone, HGH ramps up significantly in adolescence, peaks between age twenty and thirty, then drops precipitously. Very low HGH levels can cause a host of negative effects: higher total and bad cholesterol; lower good cholesterol; less muscle tone, strength, and mass, more fat; reduced sports performance; and decreased cognition. No wonder it's such an easy sell to middle-aged men who feel they're losing a step.

In the body, HGH is manufactured by the anterior pituitary gland at the base of the brain, and it is secreted in pulses throughout the day. In a lab, it's derived from E. coli bacteria or mouse cell lines in a form that is "bioidentical," or chemically indistinguishable from the stuff your brain pumps out. In order to work, you need to inject it regularly into your calves, glutes, or thighs—once a day being standard protocol.

Like testosterone, it seems to "work" in a broad sense, though each person's response to injected HGH is unique. Some report improved complexion and eyesight, less fat, and more energy, muscle mass, and capacity to exercise; others feel and see very little difference.

Downsides? Expense, for one. You'll shell out about $750 per month for the normal regimen—assuming you're taking it legally, under a doctor's supervision. Go rogue, and who knows what you'll wind up taking—or how many years in the slammer you'll get for trafficking in illegal medications if you're caught (usually about five). Controlled doses of HGH are relatively safe. Some people report short-term temporary disruptions in their blood sugar regulation. However, taking too much over a long period of time may start to give you that suave Neanderthal look that women love so much: the big brow, big jaw, and big hands evident on Barry Bonds after his years on performance-enhancing drugs. It's not a look that's terribly popular on singles night. Plus, it's permanent, and the effects of taking too much HGH can ultimately lead to kidney failure, heart disease, high blood pressure and diabetes—just the kind of age-related problems you're trying to stave off.

Want a completely free, totally natural HGH boost that comes with zero negative side effects? Hit the gym and hit the sack. Studies show that both aerobic exercise and resistance training result in an exercise-induced growth hormone response—known as an EIGR—as long as you work intensely for at least ten minutes. The biggest natural hit of HGH, however, occurs while you're sleeping—so if you're skimping on Zs, you're skimping on HGH as well. Yet another reason to get your seven to eight hours in!

TABOO TO LEGIT

Like pro athletes, we New Primers want to stay sharp, competitive, and on top of our game. And we, too, have mortal bodies that can feel like they're limiting us. Most of us aren't as strong or fast as we used to be, and many of us are more prone to injury than we were in our youth.

We're changing on the inside too: after about age thirty, production of T drops 1 percent per year (one large study of healthy men found that men over seventy had barely over half the mean testosterone of men under forty). This drop appears to occur right about the time most men start to experience a drop-off in sex drive, energy, capacity to concentrate, muscle mass, and athletic performance. Drug companies have encouraged the implicit connection between declining T and decreasing performance at this age in a man's life by coining the words *manopause* and *andropause* to describe it (see the box "Andropause: Real or Imagined?" later in this chapter).

Whether these two things are in fact linked is an open question.

Through an impressive PR sleight of hand, the antiaging industry has managed to chip away at the taboo against testosterone use, beginning by referring to it as "testosterone supplementation," "testosterone replacement therapy," or, more nebulously, "hormonal optimization." Many guys may remember the ads for the Las Vegas–based antiaging clinic Cenegenics, featuring Dr. Jeffrey Life, the balding septuagenarian GP with the incongruously muscular and ripped physique of an Olympic gymnast. The large print in these ads talked about workouts and nutrition; the small print talked about "optimizing" hormones.

As the language around supplemental T was changing, high-profile voices also came out in support of "casual" T use. In 2013, Charles Staley, a highly respected and sought-after fitness coach (who also happens to be over fifty), wrote an article for the online magazine *T Nation* saying that older lifers, as a matter of course, should "restore optimal testosterone levels":

> I'm not talking about steroids here, which are expensive, illegal, and potentially danger-ous. I'm referring to Testosterone replacement therapy (TRT), which is legal, medically supervised, safe, and a lot easier to do than most guys think.

Staley's article signaled a tidal shift. Suddenly a well-regarded fitness expert—a guy who preaches clean living, good eating, and hard work—was giving the thumbs-up to supplemental T for health-minded older guys.

Just as Viagra helped usher in a new acceptance of and willingness to discuss ED, testos-terone replacement therapy has helped bring "low T" into common parlance. Google it, and nearly half a billion sites pop up (the first of which are, invariably, ads for prescription T). Media stories and symposia on problems associated with low T are ubiquitous. At one such event, Dr. Larry I. Lipshultz, a professor of urology, warned, "Right now the prevalence of low testosterone is approximately 39 percent for men over 45, which translates to close to 14 million men in the United States."

At the same time, ads for prescription testosterone products like Axiron, AndroGel, Androderm, Testim, and Fortesta are ubiquitous: since 2009, marketing of T drugs is up 3,000 percent. "Pump up your T!" one ad for an aerosol version of the drug cleverly exhorts us. "Power, performance, passion!" proclaims another. "You may qualify for a free testosterone test!" promises yet another (I did—simply by inputting my age and checking a box that said I had "low energy"). All the ads feature virile, stubbly guys doing virile, stubbly things like brandishing power tools and driving speedboats.

The marketing blitz is working brilliantly: from 2001 to 2011, the number of testoster-one prescriptions written in the United States increased tenfold, and online pharmacies in Canada, many catering to Americans, issued millions more. The taboo has been lifted, and the floodgates have opened. T seems to be the cure for all our problems. But is it really?

LOW T . . . OR BAD CHOICES?

Most men have a total, or serum, testosterone level that falls between 300 and 1,000 ng/dL (that's in nanograms per deciliter of blood, for the nerdishly inclined out there).

It doesn't take a physician to see that that's a pretty huge window. One man could have a T level that's 400 percent of another and both could still be considered normal—and feel normal as well.

One solid, supersuccessful guy I know—a celebrity whose name and face you'd recognize—has T levels that barely move the needle. But he's a lean, muscular, energetic guy, and a gifted athlete—with a wife and two amazing little girls to boot. Perhaps his estrogen is microscopically low; perhaps he has low cortisol. It doesn't matter; it's just the way his system works. On the flip side, artificially enhanced high T is no guarantee to happiness, health, or effectiveness in the world, either—just ask your average retired WWF athlete or NFL player. So in many ways, your T number (like, say, your weight) is actually pretty meaningless. You can feel great *or* lousy with T on the higher end and the lower end of the scale.

Ultimately, hormones don't operate in a vacuum, which helps explain why men are able to thrive and feel great at such varying levels of T. Hormones balance one another out to keep you on an even keel. One hormone makes you sleep, another wakes you up; one makes you hungry, another tells you you're full; and so on. As a whole, your endocrine system works like an orchestra of skilled musicians, each one responding subtly to the actions of the others and to the movements of the group as a whole. Boost any one hormone artificially, and a cascade of other hormones rushes in to compensate for the imbalance.

Given both the wide range of healthy T levels and the delicate balance of every man's individual hormone levels, testosterone therapy is an exceedingly broad brush when it comes to treating common physical and psychological symptoms. It's a generalized, one-size-fits-all solution to what are extremely individual problems that stem from our individual inheritance and environment. Prescribed for such conditions, T therapy is the equivalent of tossing a hand grenade into the midst of that well-coordinated hormonal orchestra and expecting it to perform better.

On top of that, virtually every symptom that the antiaging industry tells us is due to low T can be (and most likely is) caused by our epigenetics—those myriad environmental and behavioral factors that interact with our DNA, profoundly influencing our health and outlook. As the following table shows, symptoms like weight gain, depression, and low sex drive can have so many different causes that pointing to low T as a scapegoat starts to make very little sense:

"Low T" Symptom	Possible Environmental/ Behavioral Causes	First-Line Solution
Weight gain	Poor diet, lack of exercise, sedentary job or lifestyle, age-related loss of muscle mass, drinking, poor sleep, environmental toxins	Smarter food choices; regular, intense exercise; stand-up desk and lifestyle; time management; better sleep patterns
Erectile dysfunction	Abdominal fat, stress, relationship problems, smoking, alcohol, fatigue, poor sleep, performance anxiety	Weight loss, de-stressing techniques, time management to allow better sleep and connection with partner
Low sex drive	Stress, poor communication, depression, lack of self-esteem, obesity	De-stress, counseling, connection, exercise, smarter dietary choices, weight loss
Irritability	Stress, lack of connection, relationship strain, poor diet, smoking, consumption of alcohol	De-stressing techniques, counseling, connection with spouse and friends, socializing, reevaluating life goals
Low energy	Lack of investment in career, lack of passion and wholeheartedness in work or relationships, lack of exercise	Reinvestment in aspects of life that excite and enthrall you, greater passion and commitment to family and job, potential life change
Bone loss	Lack of intense exercise, poor diet, lack of sunlight, poor vitamin D levels	High-impact exercise, calcium-rich foods, vitamin D supplementation

As Dr. Jeffrey Bland points out in *The Disease Delusion*, the medical model we now use was built around the process of diagnosing discrete diseases with discrete causes and prescribing single-action medications, like vaccines, to fix them. For communicable diseases like typhus and polio, this works brilliantly. For chronic diseases with multiple causes, like depression and diabetes, it's much less effective.

In the case of low T, the "disease" isn't discrete at all, but instead is often the result of a series of reflexive habits that, given time and focus, you can change. Before you fill your T prescription, know that the symptoms of low T—and quite possibly low T itself—may not be the problem at all but a symptom of a larger physical, emotional, or psychological problem you need to address.

Just as men afflicted with ED in the early 2000s eventually found that Viagra wouldn't fix their failing marriages or better their communication with their partners, so artificially enhanced serum testosterone won't find you a new career, put new life into a loveless marriage, or fix a relationship with a son or daughter. Low energy, low T, and all these other problems are very often beacons in a complex network of physiological indicators signaling a system in distress. I'll readily admit that it may be tougher to address those problems than to take a few injections or to wear a patch now and then—and I realize that many of the "first-line solutions" in the previous table aren't exactly easy fixes. But they very often address the true cause of the problem.

Rather than gloss these issues over with a quick-fix solution like supplemental T, it's up to *you*, the individual, to find and fix those problems so you can move on with your life, and truly make these years Your New Prime.

ANDROPAUSE: REAL OR IMAGINED?

Around age fifty-one, women experience a shutdown of the reproductive system called menopause that can bring with it a familiar range of symptoms, including mood swings, changes in sexual desire, hot flashes, and other delights that many of us will witness firsthand in our wives and girlfriends if we haven't already.

Around the same time, many men experience similar symptoms—changes in mood, sexual functioning and potency, even hot flashes—that can appear to be a male version of menopause. Some people even give this time-of-life change a name: *andropause*. Is this new term warranted?

Proponents say yes, pointing to a condition called hypogonadotrophic hypogonadism. In healthy males, a drop in circulating testosterone causes the hypothalamus and the pituitary gland (both in the brain) to release the hormones GnRH and LH, which essentially give your nuts a swift (painless) kick, causing them to ramp up the production of T. However, as we get older (starting in our early forties), GnRH and LH aren't released as readily when our T is low. When all three hormones—testosterone, GnRH and LH—are low, it leads to hypogonadotrophic hypogonadism (I'll just call it *hypo-hypo* from here on. I just made that up, but it's easier to type).

If T falls unchecked below a certain point, eventually GnRH and LH get it in gear and supply your testes with the stimulus they need to make more T. The boost they provide, however, is short-lived: eventually, T remains low *despite* high GnRH and LH—

and that's when you get what some clinicians are now calling andropause, a hormonal shift that does in fact mirror what women undergo in menopause.

Here's the difference: unlike women, men maintain the ability to reproduce late into life, even past the point of hypo-hypo. Most of the time, the drop in T is not a precipitous cessation, as is a woman's hormonal shift, but a gradual decline that takes place over many decades. Though the hypo-hypo hormonal shift will occur in most men *at some point*, an early drop is not a sign of a permanent change. There are, in fact, many proactive steps most men can take to boost testosterone at virtually any point in their lives—steps that are outlined in the previous chapter.

The acronyms ADAM ("androgen decline in aging males") or PADAM ("partial androgen decline in aging males") are probably more accurate than a term that equates a gradual downward trend in male hormonal levels with the much faster drop, and more drastic change, that takes place in women's bodies around the same age.

Maybe I'm nitpicking, but the words we use to describe our experiences have power. They make us see ourselves, and thus behave, in particular ways. To me, *andropause* sounds like a change that's unavoidable, irreversible, and drastic. The word itself literally means an end to manhood. If you believe that, how much more likely are you to think it's all over for you—professionally, personally, sexually—and that your best days are behind you?

We all know that's not true. Let's free ourselves from the myth of andropause and start taking proactive steps to turn things around for ourselves naturally.

T: WORTH THE HYPE?

As I mentioned in the last chapter, the average man's testosterone is 25 percent lower today than it was in the 1980s, due to factors that appear to be both environmental and individual. Doctors define hypogonadism (low testosterone) as a condition in which the testosterone level drops beneath a certain limit *and* causes noticeable symptoms, including, but not limited to:

- low sex drive
- infertility
- erectile dysfunction
- fatigue and low energy
- difficulty concentrating
- depression
- irritability

- low sense of well-being
- weight gain
- loss of muscle mass and strength
- slowed rate of facial hair growth
- hot flashes, sweats
- increased likelihood of obesity, diabetes, high blood pressure, and high cholesterol

Significantly, no one really agrees on how low your T must drop to be categorized as hypogonadism—and as pointed out earlier, all of these symptoms can have myriad causes other than low T.

Regardless, the T industry wishes to prescribe as much testosterone as possible. Recently it's been found that 25 percent of men who are given the drug are never tested for low T at all, and it's unclear whether the remaining 75 percent had levels low enough to warrant therapy. Antiaging clinics also notoriously schedule testing appointments for 3:00 p.m.—the time of day when most men's T levels are at their lowest. (The traditional time for doctors to test for low T is in the morning, when one's levels are at their peak.)

Some amount of drop-off in T is expected with age, but in truth, many factors can cause T levels to decline, including:

- injury to the testicles
- testicular cancer, or treatment for testicular cancer
- hormonal disorders
- HIV/AIDS
- chronic liver or kidney disease
- pituitary disorders
- inflammatory diseases
- type 2 diabetes
- obesity
- opioid pain medications and glucocorticoids (like prednisone)
- sickle-cell disease
- alcoholism (particularly consumption of beer)
- stress
- lack of sleep
- BPA (a chemical often found in plastics)
- soy in the diet
- lack of exercise
- sedentary lifestyle

Glance over that list again. With the exception of serious conditions like HIV and testicular cancer, many of us encounter a host of these root causes—environmental, behavioral, and otherwise—on a daily basis. They're woven into the fabric of our everyday lives. So arguably, the trend toward substantially lower T in men reflects a bigger trend toward a sedentary, stressed-out, sleep-deprived, overfed-but-nutrient-deprived lifestyle.

The million-dollar question that the supplemental T industry doesn't want us to ask is: *Are we fat, sleep-deprived, depressed, and diabetic because we have low T? Or is our T low because we're fat, sleep-deprived, depressed, and diabetic?* In most cases, the only honest answer to this question is *we don't know.* Just as high or normal T can be both a cause and an effect of excellent health, low T can be a cause and an effect of poor health.

If you're truly, measurably hypogonadal—your T is low and you are experiencing symptoms that are interfering with your career and relationships—then you have a condition that requires legitimate treatment by a physician. But the rest of us—those of us who have gained a few pounds here and there and may be feeling stressed-out, depressed, or uninspired—would be much better served by going to the local gym than to the nearest "antiaging" clinic and jumping on the T train.

Quick analogy: If you've ever visited Los Angeles, you've probably encountered a Scientology evangelist or two, who ply unsuspecting passers-by with questionnaires asking if you ever "feel awkward in public," or "experience feelings of anxiety," or "feel run-down." If you answer yes to any of the questions—which everyone does, since awkward public moments and anxiety and fatigue are part and parcel of being alive—the solution they offer is Scientology. Ads for depression medication strike a similar note: *Do you sometimes feel down? Do you get the blues?* With the exception of clinically hypogonadal men who genuinely need prescription T to function, the current trend to prescribe testosterone at the virtual drop of a hat reminds me of this same brand of hucksterism: an ill-defined, made-up solution to an ill-defined problem.

ESTROGEN: A TROUBLING PRECEDENT

Years ago, estrogen was marketed as the fountain of youth for women entering and passing through middle age. Literature on the drug promised a reduction of menopausal symptoms and the prevention of osteoporosis and colon cancer. Like testosterone today, it seemed to be a harmless solution to a common problem, and doctors began prescribing it liberally.

Now that decades of data have been collected on women taking estrogen (commonly alongside the hormone progestin), the drug has increasingly been associated with a greater risk of strokes, blood clots, gallstones, ovarian cancer, dementia, and urinary incontinence.

The benefits, many women have decided, are simply not worth the many risks.

At present, few clinical trials of T extend past three years, leading some physicians to rightly question whether the current run on supplemental T may be a repeat of what happened with prescription "E" all those years ago. The short answer is that our generation is the guinea pig for an unproved and overprescribed threat to our masculinity.

WHAT SUPPLEMENTAL T WILL AND WON'T DO

Surf around on a few websites advertising prescription T (there are lots of them out there), and what do you see? Plenty of virile-looking middle-aged men staring thoughtfully into the middle distance. A few women looking at them with a practiced mix of concern and lust (*However will he satisfy me?* she seems to be thinking.) A list of the symptoms of low T (or manopause, or andropause). You may even see the results of a study or two confirming that the drug in question does indeed boost testosterone. On the site for AndroGel, the current bestseller among T-replacement gels, I found this quote:

> In a clinical study of 274 men who had Low Testosterone, some used AndroGel 1.62% and some used placebo. Of the men who used AndroGel 1.62% once daily for 16 weeks, 82% had their testosterone levels returned to normal compared to 37% of those who used placebo.

In other words, the drugs *work* in that they raise your T levels (though in this case a placebo appears to work pretty well too). But does AndroGel give its users more energy, amp up their sex drive, and make them stronger, more muscular, more virile? Does it give them stronger, more frequent erections? Will it, in fact, turn them into the paragons of masculinity they're hoping to become?

The site, wisely, makes no explicit claims about any of these things. At best, the companies tap-dance around the issue with qualified statements, buried several clicks deep in the site, like "may increase" and "could improve." Why are they so circumspect? *Because prescription T may or may not do any of the things we hope it will.*

Let's take the claims for supplemental T one at a time:

"T Will Boost My Sex Drive and Performance"

It *can* be true that supplemental T will boost your sex drive and performance, if your testosterone is actually low and you are experiencing a dip in libido as a result. A 2007 German study concluded that there was a "consistent but weak positive effect of testosterone on sexual functioning" in hypogonadal men taking supplemental testosterone. But in men with normal levels of T, supplementation doesn't appear to do much for sex drive. And when it comes to sexual performance, a 2003 study published in the *Journal of the American Geriatrics Society* found that supplemental testosterone did *not* reliably improve sexual functioning in older men with normal or slightly low T levels.

This may result from the hormonal system of checks and balances. When you flood your system with lots of testosterone, your body converts a portion of it to estrogen, the female hormone (that's why so many male bodybuilders develop gynecomastia, or "man boobs," on top of their overbuilt pecs). Higher estrogen may dampen *or* raise your sex drive—it all depends on how your system responds.

More T, it seems, isn't always better, especially when it comes from a needle (or a patch, or a pill). And the indiscriminate use of T can be seriously bad news. Many East German athletes from the 1976 and 1980 Olympics who were unwittingly given testosterone as part of their training regimen are still suffering from the ill effects today.

"T Will Improve My Mood"

One of the biggest claims you'll hear about T is that it lifts you out of the doldrums. But here again, the actual findings aren't clear-cut. One 2004 study of young men taking a round of supplemental T found that the effects of 1,000 milligrams of a T solution produced "detectable *but minor* mood changes" (my emphasis). On the positive side, the subjects reported feeling less fatigue and inertia; on the negative side, they and their partners also reported more anger and hostility. Overall, however, the study concluded that the psychological effects of T on these young men were "limited." (The wording in the study suggests that the researchers were hoping that T would have no psychological side effects so it could be green-lighted for other uses.)

A 2008 review study summarized the findings on T's effect on mood as follows: "Most [studies] do not support testosterone as a broadly effective antidepressant, but it may be effective in carefully selected populations, such as hypogonadal men, antidepressant-resistant men, men with early onset depression, and/or HIV-infected men."

The upshot: although low T can bum you out, artificially enhanced, super-high T doesn't make you super-happy.

"T Will Make Me Stronger"

Surprisingly, the jury is also still out on whether T will make you stronger. T does seem to increase muscle mass, decrease fat mass, and improve bone mineral density—all great outcomes if your T is low. But the 2003 study cited earlier—which is a meta-analysis of data collected from many other previous studies—found that the studies linking T with strength are inconclusive. A 2012 study supported these findings.

Strength, as many coaches and athletes are keenly aware, is as much a function of prior learning and training as it is the quality and size of your muscle tissue. Even tests of "pure" strength, like the barbell bench press or the dead lift, can require decades to perform with technical proficiency. So it may be that, without training, a few extra pounds of muscle bulk here or there won't do much for your ability to move weight.

"T Has Minimal, and Manageable, Side Effects"

One of the biggest and most dangerous misconceptions about prescription T may be that whether or not it does everything the ads claim it will, at least it's innocuous. The stuff's all-natural, so it must be good for you—right?

Wrong.

The first ten seconds of the ads for T always sound great and are super convincing. It's the rest of the ads that scares the life out of me. The pages and pages of small print, warning us about such conditions as:

- acne
- sleep apnea
- heart failure
- infertility
- hair loss
- increased risk of prostate cancer

- liver problems
- blood clots
- breast growth
- increased risk of heart disease
- worsening of urinary symptoms

My personal favorite? "Women and children should avoid skin contact with treated areas, as accidental transfer may cause unwanted hair growth."

Under the best of circumstances—like a scrupulous doctor's constant, careful supervision—the side effects of T can be at least managed. Somewhat. But let's be clear: T is a serious, system-altering drug, and more and more frequently, ethical doctors are voicing concerns about how little research exists about its long-term effects.

The worst reports suggest that prescription T can potentially do serious, long-term, irreversible damage to your cardiovascular, reproductive, and endocrine systems.

About 40 percent of men taking T develop polycythemia, or high blood cell count, which causes a thickening of the blood—which in turn, can increase the risk of blood clots, stroke, and heart attack. One study, published in 2010, found that older men taking T had nearly five times the risk of cardiovascular problems as men taking a placebo. Another study from 2013 concluded that cardiovascular risk went up for men over sixty-five who took the drug. In 2014, with these findings in mind, the FDA launched an initiative to reassess the safety of prescription T.

On a side note, a phlebotomist I'm friendly with—who has taken my blood repeatedly for testing purposes—told me that some of her most dedicated clients are bodybuilders. They need transfusions frequently, she explained, because the massive loads of steroids they take make their blood sludgy.

Though testosterone therapy doesn't cause prostate cancer, research indicates that it may make an existing prostate cancer worse, or hasten its growth. That's worrisome, especially given the mounting evidence that many of us over forty are walking around with slow-growing prostate cancer that probably won't affect us during our lifetime—unless, of course, some external factor causes its growth to accelerate.

The side effect that many doctors and advertisers do mention, at least in passing, is that supplemental T causes your testicles to shrink, and your own natural production of the hormone to shut down temporarily—or in some cases permanently (depending on how long you're on the drugs, and how much you take). However you feel about a smaller pair of balls, lower natural T production is no joke. It can mean that once you start, you're on prescription T for the rest of your life. Like those East German Olympic athletes, who are still suffering the consequences of being unwittingly doped some thirty years ago, you and your body will be changed forever. This is part of what makes antiaging clinics such a safe business proposition: unlike Viagra, which you may be able to take or leave, T can skew your system so that, now and forever, your body will need supplemental T. It makes you an addict, and that's why my four-word summary of supplemental T is that it's a "deal with the devil."

The rest of your life is, we hope, a long, long time. Are you willing to keep up with the patches, sprays, roll-ons, or injections till then? Laying aside the cost (testosterone therapy runs more than $500 a month) and the inconvenience (a safe and smart supplementation program requires frequent self-injections, more frequent doctor consultations than you're probably used to, and, unless you have a thing for bearded ladies, serious discretion about whom you hug with your shirt off). Given all that, do you really want to be unable to produce your own T, and more or less hooked on an expensive drug . . . possibly for the rest of your life?

Another great irony: by reducing and sometimes shutting down natural T production, supplemental T also *decreases* fertility. Adding testosterone to the body spurs a process that impedes sperm production—in some cases, perhaps even permanently. In one 2013 study, thirty-four men who had been seeking treatment for infertility agreed to stop taking the supplemental T they had been prescribed as part of their treatment. The result? Sperm count jumped from 1.8 million to 34 million per milliliter in most of the subjects. In six of them, it didn't bounce back at all. T has even been studied as a possible method of birth control—because a reported 90 percent of men can drop their sperm count to *zero* while on it. The take-home lesson: if you think you might want more biological kids—ever—don't touch T.

Finally, because T hasn't been researched long-term, there really is no telling what the side effects of the drug will ultimately be—and, indeed, whether supplemental T for more-or-less healthy men eventually goes down in history as a huge mistake that we could have avoided.

The bottom line on all this: *For men with clinical hypogonadism (low T count and symptoms), supplemental T can be a godsend. For the rest of us, it's a huge mistake.* Although many ethical physicians prescribe T judiciously (only after a patient has complained of telltale symptoms *and* a test reveals unquestionably low T), an increasing number of doctors have started prescribing T without even so much as a blood test, and only upon hearing of the vaguest symptoms ("low energy," "just not as excited about sex anymore"). Though state regulations dictate what constitutes low T, the sizable window for "normal" levels allows doctors to top off a patient right to the upper limit of 1,000 ng/dL—a sky-high T level that could represent *four times* the patient's natural production.

A SHOT OF T: BETTER THAN NOTHING?

So prescription T may not be all it's cracked up to be. But surely it's better than *nothing*, isn't it? If we're taking T, at least we're taking action that's guaranteed to have some effect . . . right?

Shockingly—no. A couple of years ago, the Columbia University psychiatrists Stuart Seidman and Steven Rose conducted a randomized, double-blind test on thirty men who were experiencing depression and erectile problems. They gave T shots to half the men, and shots of a similar-looking placebo to the other half.

Many of the men saw their symptoms improve. But the men who received a placebo were just as likely to see improvement as those who received actual T.

All well and good for vague symptoms like depression and erectile dysfunction—but what about the effect of a placebo on your actual, measurable level of T, you ask? Guess what: placebos improve that too. As mentioned earlier in this chapter, in experiments conducted by one drug company, just over 80 percent of men with low T who took a T gel saw their levels increase—but a full *37 percent* of men had their levels restored to normal by a placebo.

It's clear that T levels are highly variable—throughout the course of a day, a week, a life—and extremely subject to all kinds of subtle physical and psychological shifts, including the suggestion that something you're eating or doing or taking might cause your levels to rise, and your symptoms to abate.

This is not to say that prescription T does nothing. Many men will see some benefit from taking the drug, albeit one that comes with many drawbacks. But makers admit that, in order to get the full range of benefits, you'll have to change your lifestyle as well: start working out, eating better, throwing yourself into life.

So if you're going to have to do it anyway, why not just change your lifestyle and skip the extra T?

I'm not going to get into a full-scale discussion of medical ethics, but supplemental T administered in this way is a big-time gray area. The antiaging industry argues that any drop in T affects quality of life in substantive ways and should therefore be treated aggressively (in the same way that, say, acne is treated in teens), risks and side effects be damned. Research, however, reveals that therapeutic levels of T are far from the cure-all that they're hyped up to be, that the known side effects are considerable, and that the unknowns may be far worse.

POSTSCRIPT: IF ALL ELSE FAILS

Let's say you're clinically hypogonadal and wind up on testosterone therapy. Or you've tried everything in the previous chapter and your T levels are *still* dragging and you *still* feel run-down and turned-off. Or perhaps you've already been on prescription T for a long time, and it's too late to turn back.

First—my sympathies. Yes, I've now spilled a ton of ink (I'm almost done, don't worry!) discouraging you from going on T. But if you are on it already for whatever reason, fear not: there are still measures you can take to ensure your long-term health and well-being. Here they are:

Control the Controllable

T may or may not have given you the positive midlife change you wanted, but the advice on exercise, diet, stress relief, and lifestyle elsewhere in this book certainly will. If therapeutic T is benefiting you, Your New Prime lifestyle will only amplify those benefits. Even the most adamant antiaging advocates admit that T doesn't work by itself—you've got to get in there and do most of the heavy lifting yourself, both literally and figuratively.

And it is possible that, with the right supervision, you *may* be able to wean yourself off T, especially if you manage to lose large amounts of belly fat, which can be such a drain on your T levels. It's certainly worth discussing with your doctor.

Test Accurately

First and foremost, make sure you get tested! Many clinics and physicians don't issue tests—though how they can get away with this is beyond me. Second, when you go in to have your levels checked, make your appointment for early in the day—preferably from eight to eleven in the morning, when levels peak. As I mentioned before, many antiaging clinics schedule testing appointments in the afternoon, when T levels naturally dip, which may result in your levels being reported as artificially low. Finally, make sure you get a blood test (not a "spit test," which is less accurate).

If you do receive a low reading, the Endocrine Society recommends a second test for confirmation, possibly one that measures both bio-available T (a measure of the testosterone in your system that's usable by the body) and total T (which includes the substantial percentage of your testosterone that's bound to another hormone and thus unusable by the body).

Monitor Your Levels

You get what you pay for at antiaging clinics. Cheap ones don't offer frequent monitoring of prostate-specific antigen (PSA) or bone mineral density, two key health indicators that can be affected by T therapy. The following table shows the major health organizations' recommendations for monitoring these and other key levels once you're on testosterone therapy:

Organization	First Follow-Up	DRE	PSA Test	Testosterone Levels	Hematocrit	BMD	Lipids
American Association of Clinical Endocrinologists	Every 3–4 months in first year	Every 6–12 months	Annually		Every 6 months for 1.5 years, then annually	Every 1–2 years	At 6–12 weeks, then annually
American Society for Reproductive Medicine	At 2–3 months	In first 2–3 months	At 3 and 6 months, then annually	At 3 and 6 months, then annually	At 3 and 6 months, then annually	At 2 years	
Endocrine Society	At 3 months, then annually	At 3 months, then annually	At 3 months, then per routine guide-lines	At 3 months	At 3 months, then annually	At 1–2 years	
European Association of Urology	At 3 months	At 3 and 6 months, then annually	At 3 and 6 months, then annually		At 3 months, then annually	Every 1–2 years	

BMD: Bone mineral density
DRE: Digital rectal exam
PSA: Prostate-specific antigen

Reprinted from Manuel Alsina and Leilani St. Anna, "How Should We Monitor Men Receiving Testosterone Replacement Therapy?," *Journal of Family Practice* 59, no. 12 (December 2010): 711–12.

Note that most of these organizations don't recommend testing lipid levels, liver function, *or*, interestingly, testosterone levels. The Endocrine Society, however, recommends that the goal of T therapy should be to raise levels to the "mid-normal range," as monitored throughout your treatment. Don't let your clinic sell you on anything more.

You should definitely get your bone mineral density, PSA, and hematocrit tested, and have a digital rectal exam (sorry, fellas) soon after you go on T. Then have them done regularly—at least once a year—after that. Some doctors recommend a full prostate biopsy prior to initiating T therapy and to have your estrogen levels monitored as well, since T can profoundly affect estrogen levels. Discuss these options with your doctor.

Don't be a tough guy—these aren't tests you want to put off. Be a smart patient, and if your clinic doesn't adhere to a testing schedule that looks like the ones in the previous table, walk away. Saving a few bucks on your testosterone replacement therapy is a bad reason to jeopardize your long-term health.

PART II

FUEL AND FLAME

Nutrition and Exercise

CHAPTER 3

Fuel for Your New Prime

Nutrition

The doctor of the future will no longer treat the human frame with drugs, but rather will cure and prevent disease with nutrition.

—THOMAS EDISON, 1902

Health is a state of complete physical, mental, and social well-being, and not merely the absence of disease or infirmity.

—WORLD HEALTH ORGANIZATION, 1948

First, the bad news.

Unless you're a longtime smoker, the number one most challenging lifestyle change you'll probably ever make is to improve the way you eat. Why do you think new diet books come out by the truckload every New Year's Day, each promising an easy, rapid, profound transformation by eating delicious food you'll love and never going hungry? If it were easy, everyone would have done it by now.

I'm not going to sugarcoat this: discarding bad eating habits and taking on better ones is tough, especially when you're a few miles down the road of life, maybe set up with a life partner and kids (whose lives will also be affected by your new and different food choices), and carrying excess weight that seems to have taken up permanent residence around your middle.

Then there are your favorite restaurants, your favorite celebration foods, your favorite vacation and getaway sports, your favorite dive haunts—almost all of which come with food choices that may or may not be in line with the new habits you're trying to create. It may be easy enough to make changes when you're living on your own, but who can say no to "Come on, Dad, let's go have a burger"?

If you're the guy who goes out for beer and hot wings with the guys every Sunday, or who regularly whips up a giant homemade meat-lover's pizza for his family, or who can be counted on to wolf down the last slab of lasagna at any potluck—well, who are you if you decide to *stop* being that guy? It's another layer of meaning to the old "you are what you eat" saying: depending on where you're starting from, changing your eating habits can involve changing so many other behaviors that embarking on a new diet can amount to a top-to-bottom life change.

So I'm going to respectfully disagree with any book, doctor, or guru who claims that eating in a healthy way is easy and fun and effortless. Maybe it is for *them*—those virtuous folks who have already arranged their lives to make it possible to eat in the latest Paleo-8/16-macrobiotically balanced way (recruiting others around them to the cause, seeking out restaurants that serve what their bodies need, knowing which grocery stores sell the healthiest options). But if you're one of the many middle-aged guys who still struggle to make healthy eating choices, it's a different story.

PLENTIFUL BUT POISONOUS

Why is eating healthy so challenging? It's because in our current environment, it takes *effort*.

Back when we were roaming the plains hunting for woolly mammoths, eating healthy was simple: bend down, grab edible plant, eat. Slay large beast, cook around campfire, eat. We had no choice, except not eating, which was forced on us from time to time.

These days, the default way of eating for a middle-aged guy—the equivalent of picking up those edible plants or hacking off that chunk of meat—is atrocious. Convenient, fast, engineered-to-be-delicious stuff is everywhere. Billions of dollars are spent to ensure that whenever you get the slightest bit hungry, something crunchy, delicious, addictive, and god-awful for you is never less than a city block or two away. No time to make breakfast? Grab a Cinnabon. Peckish at 10:30 a.m.? Take the elevator downstairs for a Frappucino and a pastry. Need to grab a late lunch? A burger and some steak fries are ten minutes away. Or just power through the lunch hour on coffee and treats from the candy jar—dinnertime isn't that far away, after all. By then, you're starving, and out with friends, so you figure you may as well treat yourself to a 42-ounce porterhouse, a baked potato, a few glasses of wine, and a massive dessert.

Due credit, some places are coming up with healthier alternatives. But those are still the fast and easy choices that our overstressed and overscheduled lives are funneling us into making every day.

So instead of pretending that this will be easy, let's admit that the odds are stacked against us. Food choices don't happen in a vacuum—they're a result of innumerable factors that are, by this point, tightly woven into the fabric of our lives. We're holed up in the New Prime foxhole, trying to fight our way back to better health. But the moment we poke our head out for a look around, we're pummeled with greasy burgers and fries, zapped with chemically enhanced desserts, drowned in artery-clogging trans fats, and shot up with blood glucose–inflating high-fructose corn syrup. It's rough out there.

That doesn't mean escape will be impossible. We can fight our way out of this foxhole, picking a careful path through the minefield of crap, one nourishing bite at a time. And if now and then we take a hit—a beer or two here, a slice of birthday cake there—it won't be the end of the world as long as we get up and *keep going*. I'll be there to pick you up if you need it.

Oh, before we dive in: having said that it won't be easy, let me reassure you that eating for Your New Prime won't mean you have to transform yourself into an uptight bean-counter, tracking every calorie and carb. You won't have to give waiters the third degree whenever you order a salad. You won't have to say *never* to—well, just about anything. We're going to work on developing a kind of sixth sense for the right stuff to eat and the stuff to avoid, and we'll go for about an 80 percent success rate—which means that up to 20 percent of the time, you can screw up, and you'll *still* be better off than you are now. Of course, 100 percent adherence would be great, but I'm not going to pretend that a plateful of processed and engineered crap doesn't hit the spot now and then. Eighty percent is a tough but doable goal, and that's the sweet spot where we want to be.

In this chapter, I'm going to show you first what to do, and why you need to do it—and then, perhaps more importantly, *how* to do it. All my "eat your veggies" advice won't do you much good unless you have some smart strategies for how to accomplish all that change.

Ready? Deep breath. Look alive. Here we go.

THE NUTRITION AUDIT

1. Do you eat at least three substantial servings of protein a day?

2. Do you eat fatty fish at least twice a week?

3. Do you drink at least two liters of pure water a day?

4. Do you eat a mix of different-colored vegetables and fruits?

5. Do you eat fewer than three desserts a week?

6. Do you eat fewer than three servings of processed foods a week, including chips, additive-filled or sugary cereals, or crackers?

7. Do you eat at least six servings of vegetables a day?

8. Do you seek out foods that are rich in omega-3 fatty acids, including salmon, black beans, and walnuts?

9. Do you eat to satisfy hunger (rather than eating because food is there)?

10. Do you ever fast for more than a few hours at a time?

11. Do you eat differently on days when you exercise than on days when you don't?

12. Do you have more than three options for breakfasts that you eat regularly?

13. Do you regularly eat nuts of all kinds?

14. Do you eat less than three servings of white bread, flour, and pasta per week?

15. Do you eat probiotically active foods like yogurt or sauerkraut every day?

16. Do you prepare at least two out of every three meals a day?

17. Do you take the time to savor and enjoy what you're eating?

18. Do you consider eating an important part of each day, something you look forward to and take time to do?

"Yes" answers to the above questions suggest you're on the right track with your food choices and habits around eating; "no" answers indicate that you have some work to do. The strategies in this chapter will help you find your way toward an approach to eating that will help ensure robust health throughout Your New Prime.

THE BIG ROCKS THEORY

In this chapter I'm going to draw on the "Big Rocks" theory, which I learned about from Dr. Stephen R. Covey, the author of *The Seven Habits of Highly Effective People*.

It goes like this: Picture a large, empty jar. Your task is to fill that jar as completely as possible with rocks, pebbles, and sand (an apt image, since we're talking about filling your belly in this chapter).

What do you start with?

The big rocks, of course.

One by one, you put those big rocks in there until, try as you might, you can't get even one more in.

So then you move on to smaller rocks that settle down between the cracks. A few at a time, you work them in between those big rocks. Now that jar is looking pretty full.

Finally, you move on to the sand, which fills the remaining cracks, and voila: the jar is finally filled.

This is all dependent on one thing: *you have to start with the big rocks.* If you started with the pebbles or the sand, the jar would be too full before you got to the biggest and most important stuff, the stuff that does the best job filling the jar. Put another way, *if you don't start with the big stuff, you'll never get the big stuff in.*

When it comes to implementing any sort of plan—in this case, starting a healthy eating program—there are essentials, details, and extras: big rocks, small rocks, and sand. As someone who's always on the lookout for lifestyle adjustments that affect health, I see a lot of coverage of sand and small rocks, stuff that can make a difference in your health and fitness *assuming you're already doing everything else right.* You know those studies you see written up in fitness magazines: "Drink ice water and lose fat!" "Pomegranate juice for a healthier heart!" I don't doubt there may be some validity to claims like these, but these things aren't the big rocks. They're pebbles at best, and more often than not, sand.

Before you start wondering if red palm oil is better than coconut oil, or whether free-range organic is better than free-range hormone-free, or which type of vitamin D supplement you should buy, you've got to start eating tons of fruits and veggies every day, plenty of protein at each meal, and cut back—way back—on the chemical-and-preservative-filled snacks and desserts that are slowly killing us all. There's no way around those big rocks, and if you don't take care of them, all the superpowered, supplement-driven "life hacks" won't mean diddly.

Until you've got those basic big rocks down, don't even touch the pebbles. Much less the sand.

BIG ROCK #1: POWER UP THE PROTEIN . . . ALL DAY LONG

You may be inclined to skip over this first, and most important, big rock: protein. *Yeah, yeah, protein,* I hear you saying. In the 1980s, every processed food label proclaimed "Low Fat!"; in the 2000s, they all proclaimed "Low Carb!"; and now it's all about "High Protein!" *Message received, eat more protein, let's move on,* you're thinking.

Hold on there, New Primer. True, everyone needs protein. But you, my active, fortyish friend, need even more than most—and even more than you did ten years ago. Here's why.

It Helps You Build Muscle

As you probably know, dietary protein is made up of amino acids—twenty in all—which are the building blocks not only of muscle tissue but of *all* new tissue. Every cell in your body, from your bones to your organs to your muscles, puts protein to use. Eight of those amino acids are called "essential" because they are not manufactured in the body, and three of the essential amino acids, called "branched chain amino acids" due to their quirky chemical makeup, are especially important in muscle building. One in particular, called leucine, is absolutely essential to the muscle-building process.

An adequate and constant supply of protein helps keep your body in an anabolic—or tissue-repairing—state, rather than a catabolic (tissue-destroying) one. Like sagging testosterone levels, age-related sarcopenia (muscle loss) is a slow-moving, insidious threat to the New Primers' health and vitality. After age thirty, we lose about 1 percent of our muscle mass each year. If we don't nip that gradual decline in the bud through intense exercise supported by a high-protein diet, we risk losing our mobility, athleticism, metabolic health, and eventually even our heart and brain health as we age into our sixties and beyond.

Now that we've reached our New Prime, we can't cheat our way around these known medical facts, or procrastinate a few more years before we address them. Holding on to muscle mass, and ideally building *additional* muscle mass, should be our top health and fitness priority these days. More muscle helps us move better and burn fat, and it elevates our mood. Intense, muscle-building exercise even helps our brains stay healthy and agile. But not a single minute of exercise will do you good unless you support it with good nutrition: without plenty of the right kind of protein in your diet, physical activities will break you down rather than build you up.

It Helps You Burn Calories

We may not think about this much, but digestion burns calories. From chewing to swallowing to breaking food down through all twenty-plus feet of your intestinal tract, digestion is an energy-intensive process. Different amounts of energy are required to break down each of the three "macronutrients" of protein, fat, and carbohydrate, according to a metric known as the food's "thermal effect." Fat and carbs, being relatively easy to digest, have a low thermal effect—just 2 to 3 percent and 6 to 8 percent, respectively. But a full 25 percent of the protein you eat is burned in digesting the protein itself. So the net energy you ingest when you consume protein is 25 percent less than the total energy of the food. This means that about a quarter of the calories you consume in the form of protein are essentially "free."

Before you go medieval on a large meat-lover's pizza, thinking you'll burn most of it off in the digestion process, remember that, like any other type of energy, protein calories add up. This isn't license to gorge on six pounds of bovine flesh every night. But it is useful to remember that the calories you eat in the form of protein—as opposed to carbs—are less likely to stick to your middle.

You May Not Be as Good at Absorbing It as You Used to Be

As we age, our need for more protein increases geometrically, meaning it increases *increasingly*. A 2012 study published in the *British Journal of Nutrition* found that, whereas younger exercisers' capacity to synthesize protein—that is, build muscle—topped off when they consumed just 20 grams of protein after a workout, older men did better with 40 grams, and they may have done still better with more. Older guys seem almost immune to the negative effects of extra protein, and so are helped out by additional muscle-building fuel in a way that younger guys, whose bodies may respond more efficiently, are not.

It Helps You Feel Full

More than fats and carbohydrates, protein increases *satiety*—the feeling of fullness you get after eating it. When you feel fuller, you eat less. Simple.

This fact was borne out in a recent study, in which subjects who ate a healthy serving of protein in the morning ate three hundred fewer calories a day—with no other interventions. There was no "eat less" directive, no tyrannical "no carbs!" imperative. All they did was eat a nice serving of protein for breakfast and bango, they felt fuller and ate less. You should too.

So: How Much?

The US Recommended Daily Allowance for protein is 56 grams per day for most of us—about the total amount you can get in a handful of almonds, a cup of yogurt, a glass of milk, and a 3-ounce piece of meat combined. And that's about what many of us are getting.

But it ain't enough, gentlemen. Like much of the medical industry, the RDA guidelines erroneously equate "not sick" with "healthy," meaning that if 56 grams of protein is enough to keep a guy from *starving*, then that must be all he needs for "optimal" health as well. But a 2001 study suggested that the RDA's guidelines may not even meet those paltry requirements. When researchers had a group of older men consume the recommended daily minimum amount of protein—0.8 grams per kilogram of bodyweight, or about 72 grams of protein a day for a 200-pound man—for fourteen weeks, the men lost almost an inch of girth from their upper thighs. Since men don't carry much fat in their legs, this meant that the RDA's recommendation caused a loss of *lean muscle tissue*—exactly what we're trying to avoid as we age.

Don't assume that your GP will be up on your actual protein needs, either—he or she may still be wedded to the idea that we don't need much. A doctor of osteopathy recently tried to persuade me that I could get all the daily protein I need by eating one small chicken breast each day. He was a pale, stooped physician with unhealthy looking skin who didn't appear to have seen sunshine or the inside of a gym perhaps ever. He meant well, and he seemed passionate about his work (enough, apparently, to jeopardize his health for it), but needless to say, I haven't visited him again.

A study from the Centers for Disease Control found that, in 1999 and 2000, men in our age group wisely consumed an amount of protein well over what the RDA suggests—about 100 grams—which is good news. But it still isn't enough. Not for us.

There's a strong chance that you're probably going to wind up eating less—as in, fewer calories overall—as a result of implementing the eating guidelines in this chapter. When you eat less sugar and more vegetables, you tend not to consume as much. That being the case, it's all the more imperative that *what you're eating counts*—and that it's nutrient-dense and does something for your body besides temporarily fill the hole in your belly. Unless your protein intake is topped off, you'll wind up cannibalizing your own muscle tissue in order to survive the very slight caloric deprivation.

Indeed, despite the many cries of "liver damage!" you may have heard over the years, no upper limit for daily protein consumption has been firmly established. That's not to say that there isn't one: too much food of any kind will ultimately wind up making us fat if we're not careful. And I do firmly believe that we need to limit our consumption of red meat. But if you're an active guy, lots of protein will do you nothing but good.

Here's a good way to estimate your daily protein requirements. I'm making these estimates based on the assumption that you're strength-training regularly and otherwise keeping active as much as possible (if not, turn to chapter 4 to get started on that next):

- Take your body weight in pounds and consume that number of grams of protein per day. If you weigh 180 pounds, consume about 180 grams of protein per day. That's a ballpark figure, not a set-in-stone requirement: some days you'll down 150, others 200.

- If you have weight to lose—say 20 to 30 pounds—*subtract* that number from your body-weight calculation and consume the resulting number of grams of protein per day. So if you weigh 200, but weighed 185 when you played fullback in high school, consume about 185 grams of protein per day.

Since I don't want you to become a grams-and-calories bean counter, just try to remember this basic idea: *make protein the centerpiece of each meal, and eat about five to six times a day*. If you're an inveterate "three square meals" guy (and that's okay), just up the size of your protein serving, just as you up the size of the whole meal you're eating.

Another way of thinking about it: protein should make up about 30 to 40 percent of your total calories. So if your plate is around one-third covered with a healthy protein choice, you're on target.

Remember: stay flexible, and be aware of how your needs fluctuate based on your activities. Now that you're in Your New Prime, you need to become sensitive to what your body needs day to day rather than just eating by habit. On days when you're stressed-out, working hard, exercising intensely, or otherwise feel the need for an additional recovery boost, you may need more protein. On days when you're sitting at your desk or on the couch for long periods, you may need somewhat less. One of the major principles of the New Prime lifestyle is to know what your body needs *now* (hard exercise, light exercise, recovery, more food, less food), and to provide it right then and there.

Red Meat

Your average health and fitness nut will tell you that the key to getting all the protein you need is to eat tons of animal flesh. Red meat, in particular, has received a big PR boost recently due to the groundswell in Paleo eating; some people even advocate eating it multiple times a day.

It's a fair point. Animal proteins are *complete*, meaning they contain the full complement of necessary amino acids and are therefore good for building lean muscle. They're also easily available in grocery stores and restaurants. But I'm going to qualify the usual fitness advice and insert some caveats about thoughtlessly downing tons of animal protein—especially red meat.

Meat May Shorten Your Life Span

Although science can't pin down exactly why, people who eat lots of red meat appear to have shorter life spans than those who don't. The evidence is compelling: a 2012 study published in the *Archives of Internal Medicine* followed over one hundred thousand people over several decades and found that those who consumed the most processed and unprocessed red meat had the highest risk of all-cause mortality, cancer mortality, and cardiovascular disease mortality. An additional serving of unprocessed red meat per day—a palm-size piece of steak or a 6-ounce hamburger, for example—over the years studied led to a 13 percent increase in mortality; an extra serving of processed red meat (bacon, hot dogs, sausage) raised mortality risk by 20 percent.

It's a preliminary study, and the researchers couldn't easily sift out other lifestyle variables that may come along with higher meat consumption. But it's still convincing evidence that a lot of red meat may be related to heart disease and cancer, and may chop years off your life.

Meat Is Not "Green"

Meat is not a "green" source of food. This is the subject of several books in itself, but here are a few of the distressing highlights from the powerful environmental argument against eating meat:

- It takes sixteen pounds of grain to generate a single pound of meat.

- It takes 2,500 gallons of water to produce a pound of meat, but only 25 gallons to produce a pound of wheat.

- Raising animals for food consumes over half of all water used in the United States.

- More than 90 percent of the Amazon rain forest cleared since 1970 has been used for global meat production.

- Eighty-seven percent of the agricultural land in the United States is devoted to feed for livestock.

- Fifty-one percent of greenhouse gases come from factory farms—making the meat industry officially the worst offender in the fight against global warming.

As much as I enjoy a steak now and then, I've heard enough of this type of information to make me very selective about when I eat meat. I encourage you to do the same.

Good Meat Is Expensive

If you love meat—and if you want to remain as green as possible—you'll need to consume grass-fed, organic, free-range meat and poultry—and that means you'll have to pay two to three times what you'll pay for the factory-raised stuff.

My Favorite—and Least Favorite—Proteins

I will very occasionally eat red meat, but I prefer to think of it as a celebratory food to be eaten infrequently, like caviar. (The word *carnival* shows us, by its derivation from the same word that gives us *carnivore*, that meat has long been associated with special occasions.)

About a third of the protein I eat comes from fish, poultry, and sardines (a huge favorite, and an underappreciated superfood for men—see the box later in this chapter); the other two-thirds of protein in my diet comes strictly from vegetable sources.

The following are my recommendations for the best protein sources:

- sardines
- wild-caught salmon
- organic poultry
- kidney beans (excellent source of leucine)
- legumes (beans)
- lentils

- quinoa
- chickpeas
- chia
- nuts and nut butters
- peas
- protein powders (pea and hemp)

My Beef with Dairy

You probably noticed a distinct lack of references to dairy products—milk, cottage cheese, and so on—in my recommended protein list.

What's the deal, you ask? Aren't milk and eggs complete proteins, filled with amino acids, readily available everywhere, and relatively inexpensive?

SARDINES—STEALTH SUPERFOOD FOR MEN

I recently had a full blood and nutritional profile taken by the head nutritionist for Red Bull, a guy who looks after the likes of Lolo Jones, NASA astronauts, and Blake Griffin for a living. Twenty vials of blood were taken, and the report came back as thick as a Jack Reacher novel. Your GP gives you the CliffsNotes, but I got the unabridged, authoritative text, with nothing omitted, and I spent days devouring it.

At my follow-up consultation, the first thing out of the nutritionist's mouth was "You have the best omega-3 profile of anyone I have tested—ever. What do you take?" This was coming from a guy who supervises athletes whose livelihoods depend on their bodies working optimally—people who often have teams of chefs on staff, preparing every morsel for them. For a health and fitness hobbyist like me, this was high praise indeed. I'd hacked the system.

What's my secret, he asked?

Sardines.

I told him that when I travel in Europe in the summer, sardines are pretty much all I live on for lunch and dinner. In Greece a few years back, I consumed the little buggers for ten days straight. Back home in California, I eat a non-BPA can of the Vital Choice brand of sardines almost every day.

So why do I like this often-overlooked, frequently disparaged form of protein so much? For one thing, sardines contain significant amounts of at least a dozen important nutrients for men's health. A 3.2-ounce serving of Atlantic sardines in water provides the following Daily Value percentages:

vitamin B12: 337.9 percent	calcium: 34.6 percent
selenium: 86.9 percent	vitamin B3 (niacin): 29.7 percent
phosphorus: 63.5 percent	iodine: 24 percent
omega-3: 60.8 percent	copper: 18.8 percent
protein: 44.6 percent	vitamin B2 (riboflavin): 16.1 percent
vitamin D: 43.7 percent	choline: 16 percent

Many of these nutrients are the heavy hitters of men's health:

Vitamin B12 promotes cardiovascular health; increases sperm count, increases sperm motility; relieves depression; improves sleep.

Selenium maintains healthy blood vessels and heart health.

Phosphorus maintains a regular heartbeat; helps eliminate muscle weakness and fatigue; aids in protein formation and healthy muscle contraction; maintains libido, erectile function, and sperm motility; staves off dementia and cognitive dysfunction.

Omega-3 fatty acids lower cholesterol and triglyceride levels; prevent excessive blood clotting and improve cardiovascular health and possibly sexual functioning; increase lean muscle mass and reduce body fat mass; support brain health, cognitive performance, memory, and learning; help prevent prostate cancer cell growth and reduce the risk of developing prostate cancer, including advanced cancer.

Protein is essential for building, maintaining, and repairing muscle and connective tissue.

Vitamin D aids in the absorption of calcium for improved bone health; can inhibit cancer cell growth in the prostate; interferes with tumor growth.

Calcium maintains a healthy heart and blood pressure; aids in muscle contraction and muscle tone; helps strengthen the bone matrix.

Vitamin B3 (niacin) assists in managing cholesterol as well as blood pressure.

Iodine is essential for the health of the thyroid, which regulates energy, metabolism, and weight.

Copper plays a part in regulating heart rhythm and reducing cholesterol.

Riboflavin is important in helping muscles heal and repair.

Choline is essential for muscle and nerve function.

Most of the health benefits of sardines are even more important as you age and focus more on your heart, brain, male "plumbing," and the prevention of chronic disease. For me, sardines are a "desert island food"—the one single food I could live on reasonably well, and happily, if I had to.

Canned sardines are great and convenient—if you can get them in non-BPA cans. Otherwise, your local fish supplier may have them seasonally (February and March, particularly). Grilling is the best way to cook them. And since many of the sardine's predators—tuna and cod, for example—have been overfished, smaller prey fish like sardines are plentiful in the oceans, so you can eat them relatively guilt-free.

Acquiring the taste for sardines is easier than you may think. After avoiding them for most of her life, my wife has recently started eating them and has begrudgingly admitted that she enjoys them. Do yourself—and your health—a favor.

All true. But you pay a steep health price for those perks.

I don't mind some *organic* dairy products in moderation. But if at all possible, you should steer away from the stuff completely. Dairy products, according to many studies, are linked very strongly to prostate cancer. One compelling example: a 2013 study from the *Journal of Nutrition* tracked over twenty thousand participants for twenty-eight years and found that those who consumed more than 2.5 servings of dairy products per day were at a 12 percent increased risk of prostate cancer compared with those who consumed less than half a serving (one serving being an 8-ounce glass of milk or 2 ounces of cheese). Men who drank more than a glass of whole milk a day had *double* the risk for fatal prostate cancer compared with men who drank less.

What about the egg, that other seemingly health-friendly family-farm product? Unfortunately for over-easy fanatics, a recent US study found that eggs may increase the risk of developing advanced prostate cancer. Researchers from the University of California, San Francisco, and the Harvard School of Public Health evaluated data from 27,607 men who had been followed from 1994 to 2008 and who were prostate cancer–free at the beginning of the period. Healthy men who ate 2.5 eggs or more per week had an 81 percent higher risk of developing advanced prostate cancer compared with men who ate fewer than 0.5 eggs per week on average.

The vast majority of dairy products—eggs included—are produced on farms that prioritize efficiency and low cost over quality. As a result, a host of chemicals—many carcinogenic—are regularly found in both eggs and milk; a recent study found that 90 percent of the total estrogens in the environment come from animal waste, and that such hormones are found in animal food products even if the animals are not injected with or fed hormones. Eggs cause nearly 150,000 cases of salmonella poisoning a year, and some studies have even shown that, over time, eating an egg a day can clog your arteries as much as five cigarettes a day would. Even the US Department of Agriculture—an organization not known for its candor about its own products—does not allow any of its advertising for eggs to proclaim that they are "safe," "nutritious," or even "healthy."

So when it comes to dairy products and eggs, I advocate serious moderation. For dairy products, aim for a serving or two a week, at most—and keep it organic. If you consume milk for the taste, I urge you to switch to organic, unsweetened rice or almond milk, both of which have a distinct, naturally sweet taste very similar to milk, and which work well for cooking too. And if you can't bear to crack your egg habit completely, two per week—from organic, free-roaming, and pasture-raised hens—should be your limit.

BIG ROCK #2: LOAD UP ON (THE RIGHT) FATS

In my office I keep a tub of coconut oil—thick, nutritious, nutty, and, I've come to think, delicious. Whenever I get the slightest bit hungry, tired, or unfocused, I walk over and grab a scoop. And back when I was training for triathlons in Australia, my coach had me down two tablespoons of straight olive oil prior to getting in the pool.

Twenty years ago, such behaviors would have been considered wantonly risky, especially given my history of cardiovascular issues. "That stuff is loaded with calories and saturated fat!" a mid-nineties-era doctor would have told me sternly. "Do you have a death wish?"

These days, though, it's become clear that you can't just lump all fats together in one oily glob and declare the whole thing good or bad. The many types of fat found in common foods include some of our deadliest enemies and our most trusted allies in the fight against chronic disease.

Fats to Avoid

Here are the fats you should avoid:

Trans Fats

Originally manufactured as a "healthier" alternative to butter, these chemically altered substances—which usually bear descriptors like "partially hydrogenated" in the ingredients list—raise your level of LDL (the "bad" cholesterol) and clog your arteries, and they are linked to an elevated risk of heart disease, inflammation, obesity, and stroke. You'll find them in processed, packaged foods like crackers, cake and baking mixes, fast foods, and elsewhere.

As the bad news about trans fats became common knowledge in the 2000s, more and more food manufacturers started offering trans-fat-free alternatives. But you shouldn't be eating that stuff either, in part because another possible culprit, found in many of the same foods, has been discovered . . .

Omega-6 Fats

Like trans fats, omega-6 fats are associated with inflammation and heart disease, but unlike their partially hydrogenated cousins, which crop up in natural foods only in trace amounts, omega-6s occur in abundance in nature. In small amounts, omega-6s aren't terrible for you. The trouble is that in industrialized countries like the United States, the quantity of omega-6s in our diets relative to the quantity of beneficial omega-3s has climbed steeply since the late 1960s—mostly due to the massive amounts of processed vegetable and seed oils in our diets. A 2008 study published in the journal *Experimental Biology and Medicine* found that it was the ratio between these two types of fatty acids, rather than the overall quantity of either omega-6 or omega-3 in the body, that influenced risk of chronic disease. The lower the ratio (more 3, less 6), the better the health outcomes. In other words, it's not enough to load up on the good stuff—you also have to cut down on the bad stuff.

Unfortunately, our diets have been moving in exactly the wrong direction. From 1967 to 1999, Americans' consumption of soybean oil, for example, jumped from close to zero to almost twenty-four pounds per year—a quantity amounting to around 7 percent of total calories, and closely paralleling the sharp increase in the incidence of chronic diseases among Americans during that same time.

In addition to soybean oil, omega-6s lurk in cottonseed oil, canola oil, safflower oil, corn oil, and, perhaps the worst offender, sunflower oil. As with trans fats, you'll find many of these oils in packaged and prepared foods. If you eat these things (hopefully only occasionally), read the label carefully. Lately I've noticed processed foods cropping up with the label "Fortified with Omega Fatty Acids," without indicating whether those omegas were the beneficial or the detrimental kind. Omega-6s are also found in the feed of many of the conventionally raised animals used to make meat in this country.

Smart Fats

So trans fats and omega-6 fats are the fats to avoid. But there are plenty of good fats that you can include in your diet instead. Your allies—what I'll call the "smart fats"—are *medium-chain triglycerides* (MCTs) found in coconut oil and palm kernel oil, and *omega-3 fatty acids*, found in fatty fish, avocado, and macadamia nuts.

These fats are not only considered safe, but they're are among the healthiest things you can eat. Here's why:

Smart fats help keep you sharp and moving: Far from clogging your arteries, as was once thought, MCTs go straight to your liver for use as a fast-acting, clean-burning energy source. They also have a therapeutic effect on brain disorders like Alzheimer's and epilepsy. I usually put two teaspoons of straight-up MCTs in my smoothies, and again in my matcha green tea, every morning.

Smart fats increase energy expenditure and may fight obesity: A 2003 study published in the journal *Obesity Research* found that in heavier men, a diet rich in MCTs resulted in more fat loss than diets high in long-chain triglycerides (LCTs), and concluded that "MCTs may be considered agents that aid in the prevention of obesity or potentially stimulate weight loss."

Smart fats reduce inflammation, heart disease, and other chronic diseases: The hype over omega-3 fats is not an exaggeration. These essential fats (so called because we don't produce them in the body and must get them from our diet) regulate blood clotting, build cell membranes, and support cell health. It's a polyunsaturated fat—the type that reduces both blood triglycerides and harmful LDLs. One study from the Harvard School of Public Health listed low dietary omega-3s as one of the top preventable causes of death in the United States—attributing *nearly one hundred thousand deaths per year* to this single dietary shortcoming. A 2002 review study reported that fish oil was effective in treating chronic inflammatory diseases like rheumatoid arthritis, Crohn's disease, colitis, lupus, and other conditions. The 2008 study cited earlier also found that beefing up your omega-3 consumption and lowering your omega-6s could help "reduce the risk of many chronic diseases of high prevalence in Western societies, as well as in the developing countries."

Smart fats help you stay buff: As if the health-boosting benefits already discussed weren't enough, omega-3 fatty acids also appear to help stave off *sarcopenia*—a loss of muscle mass, common in older adults, which has been associated with loss of mobility, arthritis, an increased risk of falling, and impaired blood sugar control. A recent review study found that fish oil increases the anabolic (tissue-building) effects of weight training.

Several types of omega-3 fatty acids exist. Animal sources contain eicosapentaenoic acids (EPAs) and docosahexaenoic acids (DPAs), which are directly usable by the body; vegetable sources contain alpha-linolenic acids (ALAs), which must be broken into EPAs and DHAs to be usable. Humans aren't very efficient at that process, however. Since only about 5 percent of the ALAs in vegetable sources like flaxseed is properly broken down, this is one nutrient that's important to get from animal sources—particularly fish.

So: How Much?

How much smart fat should we get every day? As with protein, I'm inclined to say "as much as you can." Don't turn down an opportunity, for example, to eat fatty fish or coconut. But for starters, see if you can get three to six servings daily of a mix of the following foods:

- fatty fish
- coconut (and coconut-based products like coconut oil)
- hemp and hempseeds
- avocados
- macadamia nuts
- chia
- wild rice
- walnuts
- black and kidney beans
- fish oil supplement

FREE-RANGE, HORMONE-FREE, HUMANE, CHEMICAL-FREE, OXFORD-EDUCATED?

Just about every grocery store these days gives you many options for protein-rich foods like poultry, eggs, and dairy products, arranged on a sliding scale of virtuousness. In general, the cheaper something is, the more likely it is to have come from a factory that subjects animals to inhumane conditions, shoots them up with chemicals (antibiotics to combat diseases; hormones such as testosterone, estradiol, and progesterone to encourage them to grow faster; recumbent bovine growth hormone, or rBGH, to encourage milk production), houses them close together, or all of the above. The more expensive stuff comes from smaller facilities where the animals are treated better and live closer to their natural state.

I often joke that this is a kind of "guilt spectrum"—you pay more so you can eat these products with a clearer conscience. Soon enough they will guarantee that the chicken you're eating was educated at Oxford and died a painless death surrounded by friends and family, all doing a somber version of the chicken dance.

Amusing as this guilt spectrum is, I nonetheless personally tend to go for the products that are as close to nature as possible. The FDA may well vouch for the safety of meat—but I am *extremely* wary of any statement the FDA makes about food products. Since you can't ethically test a tainted food product such as hormonally enhanced beef in humans over decades to see if it's actually safe, any claim as to the long-term safety of such products is really nothing more than speculation. And I'm just not convinced that there are "safe" levels of the hormones, antibiotics, heavy metals, and other toxins that our farm animals are raised on—especially if you eat lots of protein. There are simply too many historical examples of science declaring a substance safe, only to recant when other research traces various nasty illnesses back to those same substances (read up on the history of lead in US manufacturing products for a prime example).

So I'm for taking a cautious approach. Contrary to what the food industry would have me believe, I am not comfortable with any level of synthetic hormones in the food I eat, buy, or prepare for my family. Hormones are powerful stuff, and when you throw off your natural balance with additives and growth-enhancers, you invite long-term negative effects on your sexual functioning, development, and overall health, while increasing your risk of bone loss and cancer. I realize this means spending a little more money—sometimes much more—to get protein in the most natural state possible. So generally speaking, I'd recommend this: *eat the cleanest food your budget allows.*

BIG ROCK #3: EAT VEGGIES AND FRUITS

Here's a big rock that is true—always has been true, and always will be true: Eat your veggies and, to a slightly lesser extent, your fruits. Often. Liberally. Gluttonously.

The best types of veggies to consume are as follows:

- Leafy greens: spinach, swiss chard, lettuce, mustard greens

- Cruciferous: broccoli, cauliflower, cabbage, brussels sprouts, bok choy, kale

- Brightly colored: tomatoes, bell peppers, summer squash, eggplant (all technically fruits)

In general, *all* veggies are good for you, but these in particular are dense with health-boosting phytonutrients. They're also high in complex carbohydrates, potassium, folic acid, vitamins A and C, and fiber.

Many diet plans allow an unlimited amount of these foods, and it's easy to see why: vegetables in your diet may reduce the risk of heart disease, including heart attack and stroke, and also reduce the risk of diabetes, kidney stones, bone loss, high blood pressure, and certain cancers.

Vegetables are also heavy on nutrients and light on calories, and, because of their bulk, are very hard to overeat. If you're trying to lose weight, the very first intervention I would suggest is consuming six hand-sized servings of nonstarchy vegetables a day. That's an aggressive number that seems like a lot to many people. And you probably won't have to do that forever. But by filling up on the good stuff, you top off your tank of beneficial nutrients and leave little space for junk.

Because they contain fructose—a form of simple sugar—fruits have gotten a bit of a bad rap in recent years. Sugar, of course, is linked to obesity, diabetes, weight gain, and other metabolic problems. The sugar in whole fruits, however, is *not* linked to adverse health effects—no matter how much you eat in that form. That's partly because whole fruits also contain fiber, which slows the absorption rate of the sugar while simultaneously stimulating satiety and preventing your blood sugar from spiking. It's fairly easy to eat a thousand calories of chocolate chip cookies, but unless you're starving, you'll stop crunching long before you eat a thousand calories of apples (about a dozen medium-size ones).

As you refine your diet, you may become more selective about how and when you eat fruit. But if you're starting from the "average guy" doughnuts-and-burgers-and-dessert diet, your problem is definitely *not* too much fruit. If I could convince you to eat an apple instead of a danish in the morning, I'd have a huge win, and we can worry about refining things later.

Like vegetables, fruits may reduce the risks of heart disease, certain types of cancers, obesity, and high blood pressure. Fruit is low in fat, sodium, and calories. Dried fruit isn't as beneficial as fresh—you lose the hydrating, satiating benefits that whole fruit provides—but it is fine in moderation and convenient if you're traveling or hiking. But avoid fruit juices, which, as you've probably read, are more or less pure sugar with none of the beneficial fiber that helps slow absorption.

As with veggies, eating a variety of fruits is better than sticking to standbys. These are some of the best choices for men over forty:

- apples

- blackberries

- citrus fruits (lemon and grapefruit especially)

- peaches

- pears

Get a variety, get them often. Every time you sit down to eat anything, have veggies and fruits as well. This may be the biggest rock of all.

DON'T LISTEN TO THE FDA

I don't have a lot of faith in the FDA. In fact, I trust them about as much as I trust the devil.

Strong stuff, I know. But here's where I'm coming from: The FDA's purported mission statement is to "protect the public health by assuring that foods are safe, wholesome, sanitary, and properly labeled." Such a broad and far-reaching mission requires an enormous amount of objectivity and a capacity to make thousands of clear, unbiased judgments on a regular basis, and to relay that information to the public in a clear, unbiased way.

Unfortunately, it doesn't happen. In the last few years, many top FDA officials have come directly from the multinational agrochemical and agricultural biotechnology corporation Monsanto—and have pushed for policies that benefit the agro-giant while in office. In 2012, a huge push, including 89 percent of Republicans, 90 percent of independents, and 93 percent of Democrats, was made to label genetically-modified foods—a simple, overwhelmingly popular measure that would have given consumers a means to make more informed choices about the safety of the food they ate. A million people petitioned the FDA to make it happen. One poll showed that 82 percent of Americans favored labeling.

But it was shot down. The FDA claimed, controversially, that GMOs were "substantially equivalent" to nonmodified foods.

True or not, when a taxpayer-funded organization refuses to undertake an easy-to-implement measure falling squarely within its purview—which those same taxpayers support almost unanimously—it's clear to me that its interests don't lie in serving and educating the public.

Until the FDA severs its ties with this food giant and makes good on its promise to serve the health and safety of the public, its recommendations won't mean much to me.

And this is only one example of the way in which the food industry exerts its considerable power to influence the messages consumers receive about the health and safety of its products. Back in 2008, First Lady Michelle Obama began her antiobesity crusade, sounding notes about reducing processed food consumption and getting kids to eat cleaner, more natural foods. A few years later, her message was diluted considerably to "Exercise more and eat fewer calories." What happened in the interim? Coca-Cola, Pepsi, Kraft, and other food industry giants signed on as partners in her crusade.

And let's not even get into the congressional decisions over the last few years to classify pizza, french fries, and, at one point, ketchup, as *vegetables* in kids' school lunches. As Ronald Reagan once said, "The nine most terrifying words in the English language are 'I'm from the government and I'm here to help.' "

He should know—he approved the ketchup-as-vegetable classification.

BIG ROCK #4: HYDRATE

You are 60 percent water. Your lungs are 90 percent water. Blood, 82 percent. Skin, 80 percent. And your brain, the thing you rely on to read and process these words? It's 70 percent good-old H_2O. If you drained all the water out of a normal-size man, you'd get eight cases of standard-size bottled water.

So yeah. Drinking water is pretty important.

How important? So much so that a 1 to 2 percent loss of water in the body leads to measurable decreases in sports performance. When you get into the 3 to 4 percent range, problems like increased heart rate and body temperature become evident.

Water is also essential to the fat-burning process—so chronic dehydration can actually hamper your efforts to get or stay lean.

Water is, in many ways, the perfect drink. No calories. Immediately usable by the body. Easy on digestion. One hundred percent natural. One hundred percent essential. You can drink too much of it, leading to a dangerous condition called hyponatremia. But only if you really, really try.

Drinking water should be a reflex. By the time your body signals thirst, you're already sufficiently dehydrated to cause a 1 to 2 percent drop in physical performance—so try to hydrate before you actually get thirsty. Ordering at a restaurant? Order water to drink. Passing a water fountain? Grab a few sips. Working out hard? Guzzle at will between sets. You've certainly heard the eight-to-ten-glasses-a-day recommendation, and if you need the numbers as a guide, then by all means keep track. I drink water in abundance, virtually all day, every day, and when I don't, I feel worse for it.

BIG ROCK #5: EASE UP ON THE JUNK

"Clean eating" is a powerful, healthy concept. It means, more or less, that you eat only things that: (1) grow out of the ground and (2) walk on the ground, swim in the ocean, or fly in the sky—or come from animals that do one (or more) of these things.

In other words, if you can't recognize a food product as natural, real, and wholesome—skip it.

Taking a step back for a moment, we can see that it's only within the last fifty to seventy-five years—within our parents' lifetimes—that the concept of "eating clean" would have even been relevant. Years ago, the only food options were natural, healthy ones, and the corn-and-sugar-laden junk that comes from colorful boxes was largely unheard of (the phrase *junk food* wasn't coined until 1972). That we now have to remind ourselves that there's a nutritional difference between the avalanche of artificial food products foisted on us by agro-manufacturers and, say, whole fruits and vegetables is a reflection of how firmly those manufacturers have infiltrated our kitchens, dining rooms, and digestive tracts.

So as much as possible, cut out anything you don't recognize as natural or couldn't whip up yourself from whole, natural ingredients without needing a chemistry lab to do it. If you're going to buy something with an ingredients list (like bread), *read it*: *maltodextrin* and *xylose* (code names for sugar) do not appear in nature.

In addition, start to cut out the sugar. We've come to think of sugar as a fairly benign indulgence, something pleasant to dig into when we're celebrating, socializing, or just hanging out.

It's not. Instead, it's one of the worst dietary offenders of all.

Added sugar is *everywhere* in the grocery store, and influential forces are working overtime to ensure that it stays there. They don't have a terribly difficult job: in its purest form (in soft drinks, for instance), sugar lights up the same pleasure centers as some of the most powerful narcotics, and some studies have indicated that it's *eight times* more addictive than cocaine.

YOUR BODY ON SUGAR

Wow, that dessert buffet looks good, doesn't it? Maybe you'll grab yourself a slice of pie. Or an almond crème croissant. You may as well just load your plate with options. You only live once, right?

Hold on there, Willy Wonka. Before you get started on those sugary foods, consider what's going to happen to your *innards* when you chow down on that candy bar, Pepsi, or, yes, cold-pressed juice (you didn't think that was healthy, did you?). The ugly truth may have you reaching for the fruit basket instead.

Skin: As you digest sugar, it bonds to collagen—the building blocks of the connective tissue in your body—and causes glycation, which gums everything up. The result? Jowls and wrinkles that can add decades to your face. Fix the situation by consuming lysine—found in fish and lean meats—which helps restore collagen.

Mood: You know that grumpy, exhausted feeling you used to get shortly after diving into your aunt's fruitcake at Christmastime? You weren't making it up: researchers have found that people who ate two-dozen grams of sugar in a sitting—the amount in a typical candy bar—experienced a quick hit of energy, followed shortly by a reduction in energy and a stressed-out feeling.

Weight: Fructose—found in small amounts in fruit and abundantly in many processed foods—causes energy to drop at the cellular level, leading to a lower metabolic rate and more fat storage. Keep your eye on food labels: as of 2015, labels differentiate between added sugar and sugar that naturally occurs in ingredients like fruit. Neither one is great for you—but it's the added stuff that's the real problem.

Pancreas: Insulin, the hormone responsible for clearing sugar from your bloodstream, is produced in the pancreas. Take in too much sugar and the pancreas can't keep up: your blood sugar remains high, and diabetes—or chronically high blood sugar—can result. Harvard researchers recently found that a daily dose of liquid sugar—in the form of soft drinks, "sports" drinks like Gatorade (don't be fooled!), or juices can up your risk of diabetes by more than 25 percent. The solution? Don't drink calories. Water and green tea should be your liquid staples.

Gray Matter: Sugar-induced brain fog is also a real problem. When sugar hits the digestive tract, the neurotransmitter orexin, which triggers wakefulness, takes a little break—and so does your brain. For up to three hours. Counteract the energy-sapping effects of sugar by consuming protein along with your dose of sugary goodness—or by avoiding that dose of sugar altogether!

Heart: People who get more than 25 percent of their calories from added sugar (and they're evidently out there) have a 275 percent greater chance of dying from heart disease than those whose diets consist of less than 10 percent added sugar. This signifies a pretty clear solution: ease up on the white stuff.

In its extremely misleading brochures on healthy eating, the food industry has helped popularize the idea that maintaining weight is a question of taking in the same number of calories as you burn, as if one hundred calories of a sugar-syrup like Coke had the same effect on your metabolism as one hundred calories of broccoli. Unfortunately, that's not the case. Absent fiber, protein, or other nutrients that slow down digestion, pure sugar causes the pancreas to release the fat-storing hormone insulin into your bloodstream—which in turn duct-tapes those Coke calories to your belly virtually the moment you swallow them. Whole foods like broccoli take far longer to digest and cause no such response from the pancreas. Sugar also turns off the receptors that tell your brain you're full—making you crave even more of it. Whole foods don't do this. (For more information about the harmful effects of sugar, see "Your Body on Sugar" earlier in this chapter.)

So the problem isn't simply that we eat too many calories. No one's going to overeat broccoli. It's that we eat too much of the stuff that makes us want to eat more—namely, sugar. The prevalence of sugar in our diets, say experts like Gary Taubes, the author of *Why We Get Fat and What to Do about It*, and physicians like the pediatric endocrinologist Robert Lustig, is largely responsible for the epidemic of metabolic diseases like diabetes and obesity in recent years—which have recently become a bigger threat to global health than childhood hunger. In 1980, there were zero cases of childhood type 2 diabetes in the United States. In 2010, there were over fifty-six thousand. As of 2012, more people worldwide died of complications from obesity than from starvation.

The food industry has succeeded: we're addicted. And as with any addiction, the solution is a detox, a set period of time during which you rigorously avoid the thing you're addicted to—and control your behaviors around consuming food in general so that new, better habits can take the place of bad ones.

THE TEN-DAY DIET DETOX

Overwhelmed by where to begin on changing your diet? Try these tips for the next ten days. You may be surprised to see so many tips on sleep and energy management on a diet detox list. But many of us rely on sugar for an energy or mood boost when we hit a lull during the day; in addition, poor sleep makes us more susceptible to the munchies. Conversely, the better you manage your energy, the easier it is to eat healthy.

Here's the prescription:

1. Eat only natural, unprocessed foods.

2. Cook all your own dinners.

3. Drink only water, green and hibiscus tea, and coffee.

4. If you can't understand what's on the label of a food you're eating, don't eat it.

5. Minimize dairy.

6. Choose one day for a fast.

7. Keep a food diary.

8. Eat organic as much as possible.

9. Scrupulously avoid all sodas (even diet sodas), added sugar, and alcohol.

10. Turn off all devices two hours before bed.

11. Go to bed at the same time every night.

I'm going to wager that you'll feel amazing after those ten days—and have little impulse to return to your more gluttonous ways when it's all over. But if you do indulge—on a birthday or an important date, say—do so deliberately, enjoy the cake (or the drink or the candy bar), knowing it's a lapse from the program, and then steer yourself gently back to a more structured, healthy eating plan.

BIG ROCK #6: EAT TO HUNGER

I've been hinting at this for a few pages now. Part of the New Prime directive is to jettison the habits of youth to make room for habits that make sense for a guy in his forties. But one of the last places we're willing to make those changes is the dinner table.

It seems like only yesterday when we could wolf down practically anything—burgers, pizza, desserts, chips—and *nothing would happen*. We'd wake up the next day as lean and hungry as ever. But we just can't do that now that we're in our New Prime. Our guts revolt. The extra pounds stick around. Our energy crashes.

Our bodies have been sending us none-too-subtle messages about what they need our whole lives. Achy knees say, *Stay off the tennis court.* A full gut says, *Don't take that fourth trip through the buffet line.* Heavy eyelids say, *Time to hang it up for the night.* Many of us have blithely ignored these messages for decades, sometimes willfully masking them with over-the-counter drugs and stimulants to help us soldier on. But it's got to stop. Immediately.

As foreign or as unmanly as it may sound, it's time to start listening to the messages our bodies send, especially when it comes to food: I'm hungry. I'm full. You've got to start tailoring what you put in your mouth to what you do with your body.

When you wake up in the morning, consider how you're going to spend your day. Will you be exercising hard? Will you be sitting at your desk? Will you be under a lot of stress, and will that stress be mental or physical? Will you be relaxing completely?

Right from your first bite of breakfast, what you eat should be a reflection of how you're going to spend your day. And at night, it should reflect how you *spent* it. Huge training day? Eat for recovery: protein, veggies, and healthy carbs. Relaxed day? A small healthy snack—a few nuts, a piece of fruit, some green tea or water. A few weeks ago I was unexpectedly stuck in traffic for four hours. Instead of having a big dinner when I finally arrived home, I had something small to take the edge off my hunger and went to bed. There was no point in having a big meal, as I'd been sitting down most of the day.

Unlike the other Big Rocks, this final one is a skill—something you'll have to work on and become more adept at over time. But you will. Slow down, take some deep breaths, and start listening to what your body needs, rather than simply eating a huge dish of pasta because it's Italian night. Your health, and weight, will benefit significantly over time. (Remember, this *doesn't* apply to hydration—see Big Rock number four.)

EATING LIKE A CAVEMAN

"Paleo eating" is a good idea in theory, and it's based on an argument that appears compelling at first. It goes something like this: For millions of years, we evolved eating foods found in nature. Meat. Vegetables. Nuts. Then we started farming, and in so doing we began consuming foods that had to undergo processing before we could eat them—grains like wheat, barley, and hops, and dairy products like milk and cheese. From that point forward, according to the theory, we were off track. If we just got back to eating the way we did in preagrarian days, we'd all sport rippling deltoids and six-packs, just like our ancestors did (didn't they?).

I have no beef with the basic premise that cutting highly refined, processed foods from our diet is a great idea. And I fully agree that vegetables and good-quality proteins should form the bulk of what we eat. But let's not romanticize the cavemen: they lived incredibly difficult, short, arduous lives, and they basically ate anything they could get their grubby hands on—including, as some anthropologists have pointed out (to the consternation of the Paleo crowd), grains of various kinds.

Also, there never was a unified "Paleo" diet. Some Paleolithic men survived mostly on seal blubber. Others on chia seeds. But whatever they ate, it bore little resemblance to anything you can get at Whole Foods today. Ancient broccoli, among other Paleo-friendly foods, looked nothing like the broccoli you see in your local produce department.

Finally, cavemen weren't ripped: the chiseled abs and twenty-inch arms we see today are pretty much an invention of twentieth-century exercise, medicine, and phar-maceutical science.

Our close genetic cousins the Neanderthals carried significantly more bulk than we do—but they needed to choke down about five thousand calories a day (about what you probably eat on your most gluttonous days) just to survive, and probably died off be-cause of it. Eating for them was a full-time job—and when food got scarce, they did too.

So though I agree with some of the basic principles of Paleo eating, I'm not down with it as a whole. That much meat, and that many animal products generally—especially of the inorganic, readily available kind most of us are unwittingly consuming—just aren't good for you, and, conversely, grains like oats and wheat just aren't that *bad* for you (unless you have been clinically diagnosed with a gluten intolerance).

The one good thing about the Paleo concept? It's a convenient reminder of the "clean eating" idea, which I talk about earlier in this chapter: if it doesn't come from nature, don't eat it.

Okay, gents. Those are the Big Rocks: protein, healthy fats, veggies and fruits, water, easy on the junk, listen to your body. If I could get New Primers to lift those rocks most of the time (that is, 80 percent of the time), their health would improve and their weight would drop significantly.

If these guidelines are far outside your normal way of eating—you're a breakfast-skipping, low-protein, junk-food addict—*don't try to lift all six of these big rocks at once!* Take one single big rock—the one you're most excited about or think would be the easiest to accomplish—and do it for three weeks. Hydration, for example, is something most of us can increase fairly easily, so starting there is often a good idea for many men. Too hard to give up all caloric beverages? Start by simply adding water to your diet *without* reducing other liquids—and go from there, one small, manageable step at a time.

After that, work through each Big Rock in the same way. You may need six months to implement everything, and if so, take it. If it's taken you fifteen years to develop the habits you have now, you're not going to undo everything in a matter of weeks.

THE SMALL ROCKS

Some guys will want to stop at the Big Rocks—and that's okay. Other guys will be interested in doing every last thing they can to better their health, and they will want to explore not just the Small Rocks but the pebbles and sand, too. That's also okay.

What isn't okay is to pick and choose these concepts at random, and believe that taking a supplement or two from the Small Rocks list will offset a seven-day-a-week tube-of-Pringles-for-lunch habit. It won't.

If the Big Rocks are engrained fully—you use them comfortably and unconsciously most days of the week—and you still want more, by all means move on. But if it's still a struggle, stick with the Big Rocks for a few weeks longer and then check back in with us.

We'll be here waiting.

SMALL ROCK #1: COOK FOR YOURSELF

According to a 2011 study from the *Journal of the American Dietetic Association*, eating just *one* takeout meal a week increases your chances of gaining weight. One!

People eating at restaurants consume up to 35 percent more than people eating at home, and it's easy to see why: endless bread baskets, caloric drinks a request away, huge portion sizes, and rich, sugar-laden foods designed to maximize the *pleasure* of eating—not your health. Then there's the restaurant mentality, that "all celebration, all the time" feeling you get with a gathering of friends, copious amounts of alcohol (which further disinhibits overeating), and a convivial atmosphere—all of which conspires to lower your guard.

Look, I love restaurants too, okay? So I go out when there's no alternative, or when there's something special to celebrate.

The rest of the time? I cook. Breakfast and dinner. For my whole family. I consider it a way of protecting them. By slicing up every vegetable, searing every fillet, and tossing every salad, I'm ensuring that every morsel that my family eats is loaded with heart, brain, and health-enhancing nutrients, and simultaneously free of chemicals, excess sugar, and the wrong kinds of fat that could damage their health. I'm also taking into account my nutrient and energy needs for the day based on training and other demands (see Big Rock number six, earlier), and helping improve my physique at the same time. Six-pack abs, as any serious exerciser knows, are built in the kitchen—not the gym!

Cooking is also bonding: there's almost no better way of showing your love and appreciation for someone than making meals for her or him. Washing, chopping, and handling produce, enjoying scents, colors, textures, and tastes along the way, can be meditative, and therapeutic, too. I've done it since my days on the Gold Coast, when I worked as a chef to support my surfer lifestyle. Even then I found it a relaxing way of enjoying food in its natural state and simultaneously reminding myself of where it came from. Cooking itself can be a celebration of the miracle of wholesome, natural food.

Forget the antiquated idea that men don't spend time in the kitchen. Want to know what's really unmanly? Fifty pounds of belly fat around your middle, slowly sapping the male hormones right out of you. *That's* your future if you scarf down the sugar-and-bad-fat-laden crap that's conveniently out there for 24-7 consumption. Real men cook for themselves.

Cooking at home is also far cheaper than eating out. And for some people, this one step will save more than enough to pay for the extra expense of buying organic.

I highly recommend cooking for yourself as much as possible. Yes, there's time, expertise, and cleanup involved. But it's well worth the effort you put in.

THE "HOW DO I FEEL?" TEST

These days it seems like everyone has "food allergies": Wheat. Dairy. Chocolate. If I hear one more perfectly healthy person tell me that he or she is going gluten-free—simply because it's the diet flavor of the month—I'm going to scream.

Still, I'm willing to admit that everyone's digestive system is unique; some foods agree with us, some don't. You don't have to have an *allergy*—a system-wide inflammatory red-light response—to a food for it to not go down as well as it might. And the foods that cause you problems may or may not be the ones that bother me, or your wife, or your kids, or your best friends. Sometimes foods that are quite healthy can be the worst culprits.

The ultimate test for the healthiness of a food isn't just its nutritional content but how it makes you feel. So here's a simple system I sometimes use to determine if a food—any food, "good" or "bad"—works for me:

Set a timer for sixty minutes after each meal, and when it goes off, do a self-assessment. Am I alert, focused, energized—or am I sleepy, sluggish, and dragging? This subjective measure of a food's effect on you is a good indicator of how well it fuels you throughout your day. And that's why we eat: to fuel our bodies—not to fill them.

SMALL ROCK #2: MAXIMIZE PROBIOTICS

Your gut is a veritable universe of distinct life forms—an ecosystem unto itself. From the entrance to the exit of your digestive system (especially near the exit, in the large intestine), there dwell about 100 trillion single-cell bacteria, broken up into about one thousand different types—a number amounting to about ten times the number of cells in your body. In total, the colony of beneficial bacteria inside you weighs about three pounds. Before you induce vomiting, know that this bacterial ecosystem is an important part of many of your body's most basic operations.

Your gut isn't just the processing-and-sanitation plant for the food you eat: 70 to 80 percent of the cells that make up your immune system are also located in the walls of your gut. Your enteric nervous system—a vast network of neurons that amounts to a "second brain"—lives there, too.

Keeping the rain forest of bacteria in your gut healthy and vital is key to the proper functioning of your immune and enteric nervous system. Numerous studies have suggested a connection between healthy gut bacteria and healthy brain function. With a healthy gut, outlook improves and anxiety decreases. Symptoms of digestive disorders like Crohn's disease, stomach ulcers, colitis, and irritable bowel syndrome improve. Colds and flu become less severe. Insulin resistance and inflammation—risk factors for a range of illnesses from diabetes and Alzheimer's—are reduced.

Not all the bacteria in your gut are helpful; some, like salmonella and E. coli, cause nasty, even life-threatening illnesses. A diet consisting of large amounts of sugar and simple starches is more likely to feed these destructive, disease-promoting bacteria than the health-promoting ones.

Probiotics—beneficial bacteria found in certain foods—do the opposite: they feed the good stuff while starving the bad. Fermentation, which causes probiotics to grow, has been around virtually since the dawn of man, but only a few fermented foods crop up in everyday diets these days. Some of the best choices for gut health and immune function include:

- sauerkraut

- kimchi

- kombucha

- tempeh

- kefir (a dairy source—use sparingly!)

- miso

- pickles

As with getting enough omega-3 fatty acids, you can find it hard to get enough probiotics through whole food sources (unless you're a pickle junkie), and supplementation may be necessary. Look for a product with 30 billion—yes, billion—CFUs (colony-forming units) per serving, and take it daily for immune system health and better digestion. If you're ever prescribed antibiotics, double the dose, as antibiotics lay waste to intestinal flora. And in case you're wondering, large amounts of probiotics won't hurt you; you're more likely to underdose than overdose.

SMALL ROCK #3: EAT LESS

You knew this was coming.

As we get older, we probably need to eat less. But before you slam this book shut, let me add that the more active you are, the less true this is. I've come to believe that much of the reason that men over forty get heavier is that they slow down physically—not the other way around. And there's some new science that supports me in this claim: hard muscle contractions (the type that occur when you lift heavy weights or do intense sprints) cause the muscles to secrete hormonelike substances called myokines, which turn on your anabolic, muscle-building mechanisms and your fat-burning mechanisms. Contract muscle, build muscle, burn fat. I'll cover more of this in chapter 4, but for now, remember that hard exercise has metabolism-revving, fat-burning effects that are *system-wide*—not just localized in the affected tissues.

So keep playing, sit less, stay active, and you'll be able to eat more. I've been active my whole life, I've never been overweight, and I almost never feel like I'm depriving myself of food.

If you've implemented all the Big Rocks ideas, you've already eliminated one of the main reasons people overeat: junk food. And if you load up on veggies during each meal, you'll find it even tougher to overeat, because your belly will be that much fuller. Still, if you're shooting for weight loss and maximum fitness, there are a couple of additional things you can do. These simple strategies provide lessons in how our food environment influences the way we eat—as much influence as our appetite and the food itself—and how controlling that environment can help us eat less.

Eat Off Smaller Plates

It sounds silly—and my wife makes fun of it—but the bigger your plate, the more you eat: you can consume up to 28 percent more using larger plates. Simultaneously, people eating off smaller plates and with smaller utensils also report feeling just as full as those eating off larger ones.

Easy on the Fruit

Go easy on the fruit. This is a slight amendment to Big Rock number three, but once you've cut the junk from your diet and replaced it with whole, natural foods, start to be a little more selective about how much and what types of fruit you eat.

I know I just spent a couple of paragraphs earlier in this chapter singing the praises of fruit's cancer-fighting and health-enhancing properties. And again, fruits of all kinds are head and shoulders above what most people eat. But certain types of fruit are high in sugar and cause an insulin response not unlike what you get from eating junk food. Therefore, too much watermelon, cantaloupe, pineapple, and other high-glycemic fruits aren't a good idea. In general, stick with a serving or two per day of the lower-sugar fruits listed under Big Rock number three, and think of anything more than that as an occasional treat rather than a daily habit. (For more on the glycemic index, see the box titled "Deadly Sweet" later in this chapter.)

Focus

A 2013 study from the *American Journal of Clinical Nutrition* found that distracted eating—for example, eating while working—prompted people to eat more, while focused eating had the opposite effect.

Great chefs can take a single bite of soup or stew and discern not just the ingredients but also the way they were mixed, the temperature at which they were cooked, and the myriad simple seasonings that were used. There's a lot to appreciate and notice in food (especially if you make it yourself), and it's hard to do so when you're only half focused on stuffing down sustenance. It's also very easy to fall into eating unconsciously, with no regard to how the food is making you feel, or if you've had enough of it. So close up the laptop, shut off the iPhone, and pay attention to the people around you and the food you're eating. Focus on how it's making you feel—and how much you're actually consuming—rather than on the latest ESPN stats.

Keep a Food Diary

One of the simplest but most effective interventions for weight loss is keeping a food diary. Why? Because most of us eat *unconsciously*. We don't think about what we put into our mouths 24-7, we just . . . do it. Keeping a food diary brings a level of awareness to what you eat. Writing down every single thing you eat for three days has the remarkable effect of making you pay close attention to what you consume; you may be shocked to learn just how much you're putting away. And you've got to write down *everything*: if you bite it, you write it. If you're very scrupulous about it, you can estimate portions of each item (a portion is usually about the size of the palm of your hand), including any toppings or sauces you consume at the same time.

Once you have the data, you can visit a free website (like fitday.com or myfitnesspal.com), enter your information from the three days of eating, and get a breakdown of the calories, protein, carbs, and fat you're consuming. This is terrifically useful information for seeing exactly where you are now, and thus, how far you have to go till you've instilled eating habits that are genuinely healthy.

SMALL ROCK #4: EAT FOR BETTER CARDIOVASCULAR—AND SEXUAL—HEALTH

Fact #1: 80 percent of men with cardiac diseases *also* have some form of sexual dysfunction. That's because . . .

Fact #2: the same behaviors that cause cardiovascular problems—eating rich, sugary foods; stress; lack of sleep and exercise—also cause issues with sexual performance. Therefore . . .

Fact #3: if it's good for your ticker, it's good for your pecker. Good for the blood pump, good for the love pump. You get the picture.

So why is cardiovascular health so closely linked to sexual functioning?

An erection, it turns out, is something of a hydrodynamic miracle. When you get turned on, blood vessels in your penis release nitric oxide (NO). This coaxes blood into the penis and stimulates another compound called cyclic guanosine monophosphate (cGMP), which aids in muscle relaxation. Together, NO and cGMP dilate the arteries that enter the penis, allowing enough blood to rush in to create an erection.

Those arteries are pretty small, and they have to dilate something like 80 percent to allow enough blood to get in to make your soldier stand at attention. Nowhere else in the body is such a rapid dilation necessary during normal function. It's a Hoover-dam feat of anatomical engineering, and, of course, a healthy, functioning cardiovascular system makes everything flow that much smoother.

Sexual health, it turns out, isn't just a nice thing to have on evenings and weekends with your significant other. It's also a marker of excellent overall health as well.

By reducing inflammation and improving circulation, energy, and mood, the Big Rocks outlined in this chapter will improve your cardiovascular health while also helping you take care of your own set of stones at the same time. But if you're interested in taking your cardiovascular and sexual health to the next level, there are a few foods you should add into your own personal food pyramid, most of which aid in the formation of penis-friendly nitric oxide, the stuff that turns the "fill" switch on:

Fruits: cherries, bananas, watermelon (don't overdo this one, as it's a very sugary fruit).

Vegetables: beets, chili peppers, jalapenos.

Seafood: oysters, salmon.

Fats: butter (in moderation, from grass-fed cows only), olive oil.

Spices, additives: garlic, ginger, nutmeg.

Carbohydrates: oats, oatmeal.

Nuts: walnuts, almonds, pistachios. Nuts can help promote higher T—so eating more of them means better erections. Grab a handful—particularly of these three powerhouses—and sexual function will improve. They're even good for longevity. Just don't overindulge, as nuts are pretty calorie-dense.

Indulgences: Alcohol, dark chocolate. In moderation—I repeat, *moderation*—these two treats can have beneficial effects on circulation and nitric-oxide production. One or two drinks and a few ounces of dark chocolate per day have been shown to have measurable benefits. Any more, and you'll push things in the wrong direction.

SMALL ROCK #5: FAST PERIODICALLY

Fasting terrifies most men, especially active ones.

If you're a fitness nut, you've probably read that if you miss even one meal, you'll lose every ounce of muscle mass you've ever gained and look like a starvation victim within twenty-four hours. As someone who now fasts once a week—happily—and is leaner but not less muscular or athletic for it, I can assure you that this absolutely does not happen. At the time of this writing, there are perhaps a half-dozen books and systems on the market that advocate some form of intermittent fasting as a way to stay healthy, lose fat, and improve your digestion.

As you probably gathered by now, I'm not a "dogma" guy—I don't believe that there are hard-and-fast rules, much less magical foods or diet plans that will fast-track you to optimal health. Rather, I believe there are a handful of principles that generally make most people healthier, among them variety and adaptability. You want a body that can handle many different circumstances and stimuli—not an overly sensitive system that can function only under certain highly controlled circumstances. Many of us slavishly follow the unwritten law about eating the same things at the same times every day, to the detriment of our capacity to adapt and be flexible.

That's why I believe fasting fits into a smart diet.

We evolved to be adaptable, to endure all manner of different hardships, and to thrive under many different types of circumstances—including going for long periods without food. So I believe it's wrong to slavishly adhere to an eat-every-two-hours schedule, all day, every day, until we die. Physically, it's *okay* to be hungry sometimes.

I also believe it's psychologically healthy to have hungry periods. We live in an era when calorically dense food is plentiful. It's always possible to gorge—even to go through a whole day in a bloated, overfed state, without ever feeling our body's natural call for sustenance. To me, there's something a little screwy about that. Our bodies work in cycles, and I think it's healthy on many levels to embrace the feeling of hunger from time to time, and to simply go on with your day in the face of it.

Benefits of Fasting

My hunches are, as it turns out, also backed up by science. A host of studies have shown that intermittent fasting has many benefits, among them:

Normalizing Insulin Sensitivity

Fat is a very efficient fuel. It's energy-dense, and even the leanest of us stores enough of it to keep us going for quite some time. We evolved to be fat-burning animals.

But our modern sedentary, sugar-and-starch-fed lifestyle pushes us in another direction. Ever meet someone who is so heavy that walking up a single flight of stairs made him winded? It's because, metabolically, his body was doing what a slimmer person's might do if sprinting a quarter mile: burning sugar.

When you burn primarily sugar for fuel, you slowly become less sensitive to insulin, the hormone that helps process sugar in your bloodstream. Eventually, you get permanent high blood sugar, and ultimately you can end up with diabetes if you're not careful.

Intermittent fasting reverses that slow decline into insulin insensitivity; instead, you become more able to process sugar with less insulin, which reduces your risk of diabetes, heart disease, cancer, and many other chronic diseases.

Normalizing Ghrelin

Ghrelin, "the hunger hormone," is typically lower in thinner people (people with anorexia nervosa have extremely low levels) and higher in obese people. But it's also affected by one's eating behavior: intermittent fasting helps your body keep this hormone on an even keel, ratcheting it up when you haven't eaten for a few hours, and tamping it down for about three hours after you eat.

Increasing Human Growth Hormone

Naturally occurring HGH, as mentioned in chapter 2, is important for maintaining health and fitness, and for slowing the aging process. No wonder synthetic HGH is such a standby in antiaging facilities. Fasting has been shown to bump up HGH levels by 2,000 percent.

May Improve Immunity

A 2014 study published in the journal *Cell Stem Cell* found that periods of prolonged fasting (two to four days at a time, done every few weeks over a six-month period) appeared to benefit immunity. In both mice and humans, fasting "flipped a switch" that caused damaged immune cells to die off and new ones to grow in their place.

Since reduced immune system functioning often accompanies aging, these findings have powerful implications for older men. Two to four days is a lot of fasting to undergo at a stretch, of course, but immunity may get a boost from shorter fasting periods, too.

These are some of the main benefits of periodic fasting, but it has also been shown to inhibit fat gain, lower triglycerides, improve brain function and focus, control your appetite, protect against effects of diseases like Alzheimer's and Parkinson's, and reduce system-wide inflammation.

How to Fast

I recommend building up to a one-day fast, and doing it once a week if you can manage it. Start with a light-eating day, missing a single meal or cutting your food consumption by 50 percent for a twenty-four-hour period.

Then go for a full day without solid food, starting after an early evening meal and resuming eating the next evening.

A few parameters for fasting:

1. Water, freshly squeezed vegetable juices, fresh lemon juice with a little honey, and dandelion or licorice tea are all fine in moderation. Avoid caffeinated teas, though, and don't drink so much vegetable juice that it becomes a meal. Sip, don't guzzle.

2. When your stomach starts to grumble, drink lots of water to fill yourself up.

3. Work your fasting day into your training schedule so that it coincides with a lighter exercise load: walking, swimming, stretching, and foam rolling are all good on the fast day. Doing a Spartan Race or going for a personal record in the 10K are not. I like to do yoga and take a light run. Monitor your own state to see how you feel.

4. When you resume eating, do so slowly. Have a small protein meal with fresh vegetables and salad—about half the size of your normal dinner.

5. After a few single-day fasts, try to have a fast day every week, evening to evening.

Over time, you will start to love the "light" feeling you experience during your fast days. I look forward to them.

SMALL ROCK #6: TEST YOUR BLOOD SUGAR

For decades, we've been told to monitor blood pressure fanatically. But it actually may be more important to monitor blood sugar.

Diabetes, one of the chief "diseases of affluence" that are affecting US men by the tens of millions, is, in a nutshell, *high blood sugar*. Diabetics are resistant to the hormone insulin, which metabolizes sugar, so when they eat or drink carbohydrates or sugary foods, their blood sugar can rise sharply. Healthy men should have a blood sugar level of 70 to 99 mg/dL after an eight-hour fast (measured upon waking) and a reading of 140 mg/dL two hours after eating. A blood sugar level equal to or greater than 126 mg/dL before eating or 180 mg/dL after eating is an indication that you may be diabetic.

For men without diabetes, tracking the amount of sugar in your blood can give you feedback about your metabolism, the amount of physical and emotional stress you're under, and, depending on when you check it, how diet, exercise, and other activities affect the rate at which you metabolize food. Not bad for one little measurement.

I'm not diabetic, but I've had blood sugar issues in the past, so I test my blood sugar every couple of days to get a snapshot of how my innards are working and how my diet is affecting me. It's a simple, painless process, as easy-to-use lancers and electronic readers have streamlined things. Over time, I use these readings to help me tweak my diet and exercise program. Blood sugar too high? I'll ease up on carbohydrates. Too low? I may exercise a little less and eat a little more.

It's a very useful measurement—and one I'd rather monitor regularly myself than wait to have a doctor tell me it's out of whack in a few years, after the damage has been done.

DEADLY SWEET

The glycemic index (GI) is a measure of the effect an individual food has on one's blood sugar: a higher-GI food causes blood sugar to spike more sharply than a lower-GI food does. And the higher and more frequently your blood sugar spikes, the closer you inch toward being diabetic—particularly if, like me, you have a genetic predisposition toward diabetes.

Fat and fiber, which slow the digestion of simple carbohydrates like sugar, both affect the GI of a food. Apples, which are plenty sweet, nonetheless have a fairly low GI because they also contain lots of fiber. Doughnuts—also sweet—do not contain lots of fiber, and thus have a GI that's through the roof.

The glycemic index isn't a perfect tool for predicting the health of a normal meal, since we don't tend to eat foods by themselves. Still, since my blood sugar is sensitive, I err on the side of caution and *always* go for foods with a lower GI whenever possible, and I advise all of my fellow New Primers to do the same.

Keeping your blood sugar on an even keel isn't just metabolically healthy; it also helps prevent the dramatic energy peaks and valleys that often plague guys over forty throughout the day.

Below is a list of some of my favorite low-GI fruits, veggies, and snacks, alongside a few you're best avoiding:

	Low-Glycemic	Medium-Glycemic	High-Glycemic
Fruits	apples	apricots	dates
	berries	bananas	watermelon
	citrus	cantaloupe	
	peaches	pineapple	
	pears	raisins	
Vegetables	bell peppers	beets	mashed potatoes
	broccoli	carrots	parsnips
	cauliflower	corn	pumpkins
	green beans	leeks	russet potatoes
	lettuce	sweet potatoes	white potatoes
Snacks	almonds		
	cashews		
	hummus		
	pumpkin seeds		
	walnuts		

Note: Low is 55 or less; medium 56–69; high 70-plus
Sources: Harvard, Dr. Al Sears, WH Foods, WeightLossForAll.com

In general, choose the fruits, veggies, and snacks from the left side or the middle of the table as your go-to options, and consider those on the right as occasional treats.

SMALL ROCK #7: SUPPLEMENT LIBERALLY

By now you may be able to guess where I stand on the US RDA—those recommended dosages of various macro-and-micronutrients, including carbs, fat, protein, and all vitamins and minerals that the government publishes and revises periodically: I hate 'em.

I've already been over why I disagree with the RDA on protein: it's way too low and does not promote good health. But many of the same inaccuracies could be said of the RDA for most other nutrients. And if we could sit in on all the bureaucratic tussling of the various special-interest groups that leads to these recommendations, I imagine it would be pretty easy to see why.

Even if accurate recommendations could be generated for the average person, New Primers have specific needs based on age, gender, and activity levels. We aren't average, as a group, and on top of that, *each one of us is unique.* So I think we would be particularly well advised to ignore those recommendations and do our own supplementing as we see fit.

One supplement I *don't* recommend, however, is the inexpensive, universally available, and widely touted multivitamin. If you're following the Big Rocks—particularly the recommendations about fruits and veggies—you're getting plenty of what almost all multis have to offer, and in a more digestible, natural state.

Another one to avoid? Calcium, which current research suggests may lead to increased risk of heart attacks and prostate cancer in men. Get your calcium through leafy greens or from my favorite, sardines, (at least I get points for consistency!)—not from a pill.

Instead of these two duds, I suggest you spend your supplement bucks on the nutrients that you, as a guy over forty, are most likely to need. Here are a few:

Protein

If you've run the numbers in Big Rock number one, you've likely discovered that you're undereating protein, an essential macronutrient. So I recommend having a high-quality protein supplement on hand most of the time, and downing a scoop in water once or twice a day (pre- and post-workout works well).

What's high-quality?

I like pea or other vegetable-sourced protein more than the oft-recommended dairy-based whey protein, and *much* more than anything containing "soy protein isolate," as many powders and shakes do. Look for a vegetable-sourced powder with added leucine—an amino acid missing from vegetable proteins that's essential for muscle-building.

Protein powder is a minor violation of my "no processed foods" rule—but the best such powder is only *minimally* processed and tastes good, and it is so convenient that I think it deserves a spot on every New Primer's shelf.

Fiber

Technically, if you're getting plenty of fruits and veggies, you should be getting enough fiber as well. But since fiber has no caloric value, it won't hurt you (and it will probably help "move things along") to have a little more roughage flowing through your system to clean out the pipes.

As with anything you eat, read the label and stay away from anything with sugar or chemicals.

Vitamin D3

Research indicates that more than half the US population is deficient in vitamin D3, which your body makes from food and sunlight. Present recommendations are low—600 international units—but literally hundreds of studies have suggested that we can benefit from up to ten times that amount.

Why are we so D-deficient? Well, we don't spend enough time in the sun—and when we do, we often block it out with sunblock. And few of us eat enough fatty fish or D-fortified products to close the gap. Stay on a high dosage—about 5,000 international units—until your blood levels test at 50 to 70 ng/ml.

Omega-3

Yup, omega-3s again. If you're a sardine-and-salmon-aholic like me, you probably don't have to worry. If not, pop a few fish oil tablets a day for all the heart- and brain-protecting, fat-burning benefits I've talked about at length in this chapter.

Fish oil tablets—with their fishy taste and occasional fish-burp aftermath—do take some getting used to. Keeping them in the fridge helps. And don't eat the capsule itself: toss them in your mouth, break them open with your teeth, suck out the oil, and spit out the horse-hoof exterior. Once you're used to them, the fish burps go away pretty fast.

Look for a fish-based supplement that contains at least 500 milligrams each of EPA and DHA (you won't get both from vegetable sources).

Additional Supplements

In addition to the basics discussed in the previous section, I also personally take—and recommend you at least *experiment* with—the following supplements, all of which have substantial data supporting their benefits for men in their New Prime. The benefits include improved memory, energy, eyesight, sexual functioning, better bone and prostate health, blood sugar control, and reduced system-wide inflammation. Try a few and see if you don't feel better for it:

- turmeric/curcumin

- cayenne/capsaicin

- astragalus

- green tea

- lutein

- coenzyme Q10

- AHCC mushroom extract

- vitamin E (gamma tocopherol, not alpha)

- ashwagandha

- phosphatidylserine

I also take three other supplement formulas for general male health. Full disclosure: I formulated these specifically for men over forty—but I fully stand by them and take them daily.

- Prost-P10x (for prostate health)

- PR Labs Men's Probiotic

- EveryDay Male (for sexual health and energy)

DON'T TAKE HEALTH ADVICE FROM THE UNHEALTHY

There's a good chance you've been with your general practitioner for a few years. You go in a couple of times a year (hopefully no more often than that), you chat about your respective families and the state of your career, he (or she) listens, pokes, prods, palpates, and possibly prescribes. And you listen and do your best to follow instructions. Your GP is a health care professional, and there's a degree hanging on the wall decreeing as much. So he or she must know what it takes to be healthy.

Right?

In an ideal world, the answer would be yes. But this world isn't ideal—especially when it comes to health care.

Most doctors aren't in the health care business. They don't prescribe behaviors to make us healthy. They prescribe pills and surgeries and treatments to make us *un-sick*. The doctors I know only rarely mention diet or exercise or stress-relief techniques to their patients, in part because they don't believe that their patients are willing or able to follow through with such a program. Rightly or wrongly, health care consumers have come to expect quick-fix solutions from our doctors that require little to no action on our part—except maybe to take a pill or show up for a procedure. The implied agreement between you and your doctor is that you will show up sick and he or she will give you something to make you well.

In some circles, this is changing. Doctors are literally *prescribing* exercise—writing "Aerobic exercise 3x/week 20 minutes/day" on their prescription pads and handing it to their patients, knowing that, to a completely sedentary person, almost no single behavior can be as beneficial to a person's health as exercise is. Bravo to them.

Too many others, however, are too embarrassed or resigned to bring it up, and instead they offer a few vaguely reassuring words, and maybe prescribe a pill to treat the patient's depression, or blood thinners to treat his cardiovascular disease. Indeed, they've bought in to the medical myth of the patient as a passive recipient of treatment. These doctors are sometimes overweight and deeply unhealthy themselves, and they often do little to combat unhealthy habits in the people around them. On the way out of my doctor's office recently, I passed a receptionist snacking on corn chips and soda.

Here's an assignment: next time you visit your GP, turn the tables. Look for indications of *his* or *her* health. Does his skin look healthy? Do his eyes look vital? Does he stand straight? Does he appear lean, muscular, athletic? Would you want his physique? Ask him about his program for personal health: Is he at least conscious of his diet? Does he get vigorous exercise regularly? Is he up on new dietary principles and exercise techniques?

Paul Chek, a kinesiologist and a health and fitness expert, suggests you give your doctor one simple test: have him take his shirt off. If he looks good, says Chek, you can feel confident taking health advice from him. If he doesn't, find someone else. And Chek is only half kidding.

Doctors who have a real understanding of health, not just unsickness, are a rare breed. Med school offers little to no information on nutrition or integrative wellness. If you keep up with medical news in the popular press, you may possibly know more about cutting-edge medical research than your doctor does.

A couple of other points to bear in mind when you see your doctor: Go in informed. Check your symptoms on cdc.gov (not some random site!) before seeing your doctor. Then, instead of being intimidated by the white coat and the formal manner, take charge of the room a bit. Have a list of questions going in and tick off the answers as you get them. Often doctors speak so quickly that you leave the exam room more confused than when you came in. Whenever your doctor prescribes a treatment, get all your options first. Many doctors accept perks from pharmaceutical companies for prescribing particular medications (check projects.propublica.org/docdollars to see).

At the end of the day, if your doc is more interested in plying you with pills than in maximizing your health, don't be afraid to switch to a new one—no matter how long you've been together. Find a new doctor through the recommendations of like-minded friends, or at a teaching hospital—not through your insurer, who's trying to limit costs.

YOUR THIRTY-DAY ACTION PLAN FOR OPTIMAL NUTRITION

I started out this chapter by saying how hard it is to change your eating habits. I still agree with that statement. But I also freely admit that I then went on to throw a ton of information at you about how to do just that. And if you have a long way to go with your nutritional habits, all of those tips may seem overwhelming. But as a reward for sticking with me so far, let me remind you that you're not shooting for perfection.

Not long ago I was talking with the renowned life coach Tony Robbins, a friend who I've known for some time, after a daylong meeting together. I was curious how many people complied fully with the principles he covered during his "Unleash the Power Within" weekends—three day, fifteen-hour-a-day immersions into Tony's life strategy. I wondered aloud if it was even possible to remember—much less stick with—everything he discussed over these transformative weekends.

His response: If everyone took just *one* practice from the three days—of the dozens he tried to impart—and put it sincerely and consistently into action in his or her life, then the person would achieve a massive change. Over time, he or she could be inspired to go deeper and do more, as success breeds success. But by starting with one simple, sustainable action, people set themselves up to start the process of real change.

I don't expect 100 percent perfection on day one, and neither should you. Implement what you can, even if it's half—or less—than what I'm recommending. Take small steps. You'll still see a big change. I want this to be a plan for life, not just something you do for thirty days. It's no problem if you fall off the wagon. Just get back on it as soon as you can. If, over time, you hit an 80 percent level of adherence to this plan, your life will improve immeasurably.

An 80 percent adherence to the program could mean that eight out of ten days you eat the way I've outlined, or eight out of ten meals you eat this way, or 80 percent of what you eat is on the program—for any of these options, you're in the ballpark. The people who hit that mark on day one and continue it for thirty days are the ones who will see immediate, life-changing shifts in energy, focus, and outlook. Others may take six months to get there, and that's okay too. You know yourself—pick your time frame and dive into the program!

With that said, here are your marching orders for New Prime nutrition:

1. **Cut out the junk.** This includes fast food, processed foods (how many unpronounceable items are on that ingredients list?), white flour, sugar, and pasta. If your mom wouldn't have approved of it—don't eat it. And never drink your calories!

2. **Get smart about protein.** Consume plenty of salmon, sardines, and vegetable proteins (multiple servings a day), some poultry (a few servings a week), and little red meat, dairy, and eggs (one serving a week at most), and always buy organic if possible.

3. **Become a vega-holic.** Shoot for six servings a day—meals and snacks—focusing on cruciferous veggies like broccoli, cauliflower, and cabbage. Buy organic when possible.

4. **Don't fear fats.** Increase your intake of "good" fats like coconut oils and avocados, as well as nuts (especially walnuts and almonds).

5. **Eat to hunger.** Use your own sensations as a guide for when you're full, what foods give you energy, and what foods tire you out. Track food intake and energy levels in a journal if necessary.

6. **Experiment with fasting.** Give it a try at least once, and consider working up to a once-a-week fast.

7. **Go for variety.** Aim for variety in the colors of fruits and veggies you eat, and the types of foods you consume generally. Don't get stuck in a breakfast rut: rotate through at least three breakfast options throughout the week.

8. **Take probiotics.** Consume a non-dairy probiotic food or supplement every day.

9. **Cook your own food.** Strive to prepare and cook as many of your own meals as possible.

10. **Eat smaller quantities.** Slow down, enjoy your food more, and eat less of it.

11. **Monitor your blood sugar.** Buy and use a blood sugar monitor.

12. **Emphasize low-glycemic foods.**

13. **Keep ahead of your thirst.** Make hydration a reflex, and drink water whenever the chance comes up.

14. **Examine your doctor.** Review the personal health of your medical team, and change doctors if necessary.

That's what it all boils down to: natural foods, plenty of protein, healthy fats, veggies, fruits, and water, distributed evenly throughout your day, with no room for the crap that compromises your health. I've dedicated a lot of time and space in this book to this subject, and for good reason: along with rest and recovery, diet—*not* exercise—is the foundation of any health and wellness program, the immune-boosting, energy-maintaining, health-enhancing bedrock on which the rest of the program is built. Older guys, take heed: if you're not following these rules—the Big Rocks, at least—you're undermining everything else in your life, such as your career, your relationships, and your health. Put these rules into practice, and your life will transform.

CHAPTER 4

The Prime Pump

Real-Life Functional Fitness after Forty

Even if the day ever dawns in which it will not be needed for fighting the old heavy battles against Nature, [muscular vigor] will still always be needed to furnish the background of sanity, serenity, and cheerfulness to life, to give moral elasticity to our disposition, to round off the wiry edge of our fretfulness, and make us good-humored and easy of approach.

—WILLIAM JAMES,
"THE GOSPEL OF RELAXATION," 1892

[Learning] to think like a professional fighter in the ring [helps you] perform like one outside of it. By changing your physicality you can change your mentality. Boxing can help you face any challenge, overcome any obstacle and defeat any adversity that stands in your way.

—JOHN SNOW, TRINITY BOXING CLUB, 2014

GET YOUR DOSE

For decades, the medical community has informed us that the main benefits of exercise accrue when you perform just a half hour of moderate-intensity aerobic exercise—something like an easy jog on a treadmill—five times a week. Lately, the American Heart Association has declared that seventy-five minutes per week of more vigorous activity may work just as well. "Anything beyond that," a bored and not-very-healthy-looking physician recently informed me, "is gravy."

These recommendations have spawned a thousand big-box gyms, millions of hours of "cardio theater," and just as many trips to massage therapists and chiropractors, resulting from exercisers craning their necks to watch ESPN while they pound away on a treadmill, StairMaster, or elliptical machine.

I understand why these lowball figures are in place. They're real. Ask a cardiologist how much you need to exercise and he or she can pull out a chart showing that the additional *measurable* benefits of exercise—incidence of heart attacks, metabolic syndrome, and so on—drop off sharply beyond those minimums. And if you hate exercise and are strapped for time, it's nice to know what the "minimum effective dose" is so that you can avoid dropping dead of a heart attack in your mid-forties. Something really is better than nothing, especially when it comes to exercise.

If the minimums are seriously all you can handle, or want to handle, well, you can probably stop reading this chapter right here. You know all you need to know. Tell the average doctor that you're doing those minimums and they'll pat you on the back for your diligence and move on to other topics (or, more likely, they'll just kick you out right then and there to make room for more urgent cases). Most doctors aren't focused on making you optimally healthy and vital—they're focused on making you *not sick*.

In truth, though, these minimal workouts will only somewhat stem the tide of slow decline. They won't help balance your hormones or give you the rush of endorphins received by people who exercise more often and more strenuously. They won't build much muscle or burn much fat. They won't get you to Your New Prime.

In fact, the minimal recommendations that have been in place for so many years became the gold standard for exercise almost by accident. In a lab, it's easy and convenient to study a person's vital functions while they're running continuously on a treadmill or cycling on a stationary bike; it's much tougher to measure these things while they're lifting weights or sprinting up a steep hill or working the focus mitts with a boxing trainer. So aerobic activity—and treadmills and stationary bikes—became the go-to exercise modality in part because they were easy to study. Until now, no one really bothered to ask if there might not be something better.

With respect to exercise, I'm going to argue—strenuously—that the "minimum effective dose" should be the last thing on your mind, and that the default forms of exercise toward which most men gravitate are suboptimal at best, and a potentially injurious waste of time at worst—especially for guys over forty. I'm also going to explode the pervasive myth that looking ripped and rippling has much to do with long-lasting vitality and health.

Finally, I'm going to give you what I think are the far more effective, time-efficient alternatives to the exercise systems that are out there, complete with a sample program that will take you through these first crucial thirty days of living Your New Prime—and well beyond.

FUNCTION, THEN FORM

Let's talk body image.

Few of our dads would admit that they thought much about the way they looked—particularly from the neck down. Headed out for a date, they'd throw on some Brylcreem and some Old Spice and saunter out of the house, preening like peacocks, jelly-bellies and all. Looking like a lumberjack just wasn't a high priority for that generation.

Need further proof? Grab a copy of 1934's *It Happened One Night*, and check out the scene where Clark Gable doffs his shirt. Not that Gable looks bad, exactly—he looks like an average guy. But back in the 1930s, that trim-but-hardly-heroic torso made women *swoon*.

These days it's a different story.

Stroll by a magazine rack and you'll see title after title devoted to helping guys look like superheroes. There's a big-box gym, a few private gyms, and a GNC supplement store—or twenty—in virtually every city and town in America. Meanwhile, every guy who takes his shirt off in the movies looks like he bends steel for a living. No longer are flagstone pecs and six-pack abs the sole domain of athletes-turned-actors like Schwarzenegger and Van Damme; in movies these days, even Sherlock Holmes—*Sherlock Holmes!*—is ripped.

The ubiquity of muscle in the media wouldn't matter so much if it didn't coincide disturbingly with a surge in steroid use and other potentially self-destructive activities among men. A recent survey found that 90 percent of middle-school aged boys exercised—at least occasionally—with the goal of increasing muscle mass. Prescriptions for supplemental testosterone have gone up 500 percent since 1993. One study estimated that 6.6 percent of male high school seniors had used or were using steroids—the vast majority without medical supervision.

Performance-enhancing drugs are bad enough in professional sports, where at least there are careers and millions of dollars on the line. But when more than one in twenty boys have tried juicing before graduating from high school, it's a serious issue.

These statistics suggest that body image is no longer solely a concern for our wives, daughters, and female friends. Guys are feeling the pressure these days as well, and some of us are going to dangerous lengths to reshape our bodies to conform to the new, decidedly unrealistic norm. You've probably felt a bit of this pressure yourself.

A great irony is that in many cases, the bulked-up, ripped-down look so many men covet for its association with athleticism and virility is decidedly *un*-healthy. When professional bodybuilders stand onstage in micro-Speedos to be judged on their resemblance to Greek gods, many of them are so dehydrated that they can barely get through a three-minute posing routine without cramping, and sometimes collapsing, onstage. A few have even died from use of diuretics. A Los Angeles–area trainer I know who routinely supervises the diet and workout schedules of actors for superhero roles in action-adventure movies, told me that one of his clients, famous for his Herculean physique, was so overtrained, underfed, and dehydrated throughout the shoot that he could barely get out of bed, much less perform the extended fight scenes the role required. Another actor I spoke to, who had undergone six months of extreme training (accompanied by an eating regimen that alternated between force-feeding and near starvation that made me sick just hearing about it) to play the lead in a sword-and-sandal movie, spoke of feeling so guilty about eating a handful of potato chips during filming that he spat them out before swallowing them.

Conversely, many extremely fit men—fast, strong, enduring—don't have the coveted camera-ready, bulked-up look. You wouldn't pick my compactly built friend John McGuire out of a crowd—but if you ever needed help in a real-life emergency of any sort, you'd want him around: he spent ten years as a Navy SEAL and still can crank out dozens of pull-ups and hundreds of push-ups at a moment's notice. He's a genuine, dyed-in-the-wool badass, and also one of the nicest human beings you'd ever care to meet.

But the greatest irony of all? On the whole, our dads' generation—none of whom had ever heard the expression "six-pack abs," had ever seen a big-box gym or eaten a gluten-free brownie—was fitter than we are. In 1940, the average eighteen-year-old male in the United States weighed about 155 pounds and had a body mass index (BMI) of about 22. By 1980, he weighed almost 170 and had a BMI of over 24—just below what's considered "overweight." And in 2013, the average US male had a BMI of 29—just a tick shy of what's considered "obese." Clark Gable may look subpar if you compare him with the über-worked-out movie stars of today, but he's a stud next to today's average forty-year-old. All the fitness magazines, fitness obsession, and health-conscious living in the world haven't kept us from getting steadily fatter and fatter.

I propose that it's time we started worrying less about looking like superheroes and more about achieving actual health and fitness—the kind that will help us live longer, feel better, and keep up with the youngsters. That's the type of fitness—sometimes called "functional fitness"—that the program in this chapter will give you. Looking better is a very nice (and predictable) side effect, but it isn't the central goal. Unless you're being paid well to do it, going for the extremely big-and-cut look doesn't make a lot of sense.

THE BENEFITS, IN A NUTSHELL

I don't imagine that you need me to tell you that exercise is good for you. I've heard—and I image you have too—from medical professionals over and over again that "if exercise were a pill, I'd put everyone on it." Indeed, the biggest predictor of premature death in the world is *low fitness*. More than smoking, drinking, or obesity. Exercise, more than almost any other activity, has the potential to add years to your life.

THE FITNESS AUDIT

1. Are you currently doing any type of formal exercise?

2. If you exercise, do you keep track of your progress?

3. Does your exercise program include at least two hours a week of strength training?

4. Does your exercise program include at least three sessions per week of mobility training?

5. Do you regularly use a foam roller?

6. Does your exercise program include at least one session per week of cardiovascular training?

7. Do you regularly participate in long-distance running or cycling?

8. Do you sit for long periods during the day, either at home, in the car, or at work?

9. Do you shy away from activities or gatherings that require you to be active, run around, or go shirtless?

10. Do you believe that a guy isn't fit unless he has a six-pack?

11. Do you ever take a day or more at a time completely off from all forms of exercise, including leisurely walks?

12. Do you avoid exercise due to inexperience, orthopedic pain, or embarrassment?

"No" answers to questions 1–6 and "Yes" answers to questions 7–12 indicate that you need to put some attention into at least some areas of your exercise program. I'm here to help.

I get the basic point, and I imagine you do too: exercise is good for your body. But I believe the exercise-as-medicine analogy is also flawed. To me, it suggests that exercise is something you add to your life; an inconvenient but necessary diversion from the real business of living.

In truth, the real aberration, behaviorally speaking, isn't exercising but *not* exercising—which is unfortunately how many of us lead our lives. Up until the very recent past, frequent, vigorous exercise was a necessary part of every day, whether our business was hunting, gathering, building, or farming. There was no need for "exercise" per se. Life itself was workout enough.

In truth, vigorous movement is our birthright, evolutionarily speaking. We were truly born to move. When we move frequently, our joints work better. We experience less back pain, less depression, and a greater sense of purpose. Our metabolism improves. Our muscles grow and become stronger. Our minds become more supple and adaptive. Mood improves. Hormonal profiles improve. Name the vital sign, and movement makes it better.

The human endeavor of making life ever more comfortable and cozy has led to a startling paradox: we've technologized ourselves sick. At some point in the last century or so, we made first-world living so easy that it's literally killing us.

The very recent development of being able to make a living shuttling between bed, the desk chair, the couch, and, now and then, the car or subway, is a deviation from our naturally active state. So that's why I don't like to think of movement as a cure for anything. More accurately, *not moving* is a deadly aberration from our natural, always-in-motion state. We need to figure out more ways to make movement fundamental to our lives. That's a big part of what this chapter is about.

So what benefits can we expect from frequent, vigorous exercise? I'm tempted to simply say, like Jack Nicholson in *As Good as It Gets*, that it simply "makes you a better man," because new benefits are being discovered all the time. But here are the big ones:

Better Cardiovascular Health

Better cardiovascular health is the benefit your doctor probably cares the most about, and the one that has been the most widely studied. Exercise reduces blood pressure, lowers bad (LDL and total) cholesterol, increases good (HDL) cholesterol, and increases insulin sensitivity, allowing you to clear sugar (glucose) from the bloodstream more effectively. Your ability to perform physical tasks with less energy and effort improves substantially with exercise, as does the capacity of your blood vessels to dilate in response to exercise stimulus.

All these benefits add up to a substantially reduced risk for what's still the number one killer of men over forty: cardiovascular disease.

Better Muscular and Skeletal Health

Back when our dads were in their forties, the standard advice for back pain—or most forms of orthopedic pain—was to stay in bed. This turns out to have been almost entirely wrongheaded. Yes, if you've suffered a severe break, sprain, or strain, you may need complete rest, and you should listen to your doctor. But pretty soon—sooner than you think—it's better to get moving. As much as you can.

Muscles and bones thrive on stress and wither away without it: just ask the NASA astronauts who have to spend a surprising amount of their waking hours (up to 40 percent) on specialized exercise machines lest they waste away like starvation victims in the zero gravity environment of space. Bone, connective tissue, and muscle all grow with a certain amount of impact and stress.

More muscle does more than make you look better. Loss of muscle tissue in men over thirty is so common that doctors have coined a term for it: *age-related sarcopenia*. And though some muscle loss is probably unavoidable, much of it is within your control. When you stem the tide of muscle loss with strength training and high-intensity cardio exercise, you become less frail and more resistant to falls and injury as you age.

Better Metabolic Health

Just twenty minutes of sitting has measurable, detrimental effects on posture, circulation, and metabolism. But a recent study found that five-minute walking breaks, at just two miles an hour, every hour, improved circulation and prevented circulatory damage. Another study indicated that more frequent walks (every twenty minutes) mitigate metabolic slowdown and damage as well.

But the long-term metabolic benefits of exercise really start to accrue when you work out regularly and intensely—especially when you strength-train and perform high-intensity cardio, as I prescribe later in this chapter.

One big reason that you lose muscle when you stop working out is that muscle is metabolically expensive; it requires lots of calories to keep it around. So as soon as the body decides that all that muscle tissue isn't necessary, whoosh—it's gone.

But for those of us trying to stave off fat gain, "metabolically expensive" is a good thing—we want to keep as much metabolically expensive tissue around as possible, as it's the engine that drives caloric burn and fat loss, and keeps our physiques young and healthy. More muscle, better metabolism.

Better Mental Health

There are evolutionary biologists out there who believe that our brains developed to their current level of sophistication because we moved so much: we had to remember not a single migratory pathway but the details of multiple environments, plus the skills and know-how to thrive in each one. The fact that our brains respond so positively to exercise—growing new neurons and shoring up memory stores—suggests this may be true.

The simple act of walking requires an astonishing coordination of nearly all your body's muscles: the left leg and right arm swing forward at the same moment that your right leg and left arm swing back; then all four limbs change directions and the cycle repeats in reverse—over and over again. Add jumping, running, or negotiating obstacles or uneven outdoor terrain, and the proprioceptive (self-sensing) challenges increase exponentially—all of which require the full engagement of your nervous system, brain, and musculature.

Exercise also improves mood and outlook. Says John Ratey, the author of *Spark: The Revolutionary New Science of Exercise and the Brain*, "Exercise is the single best thing you can do for your brain in terms of mood, memory, and learning. Even 10 minutes of activity changes your brain."

Better Sexual Health

In addition to enhancing body image, confidence, and self-esteem (all of which help you function better sexually), exercise also reduces the risk of ED and reduces the symptoms in people who have erectile difficulties. One study of thirty-one thousand men found that active middle-aged men were less likely than their inactive peers to have ED.

Men with benign prostatic hyperplasia (BPH) who exercised saw their urinary tract symptoms reduced by half. Semen quality also improves with exercise and gets worse when you're sedentary.

Finally, sex is easier (and thus more fun) when you're fit: even missionary position requires some muscular strength—and the more you have, the less you need to worry about straining or popping something midcoitus. Which is a serious mood-killer.

Less Inflammation

Inflammation can thicken your blood vessels as you age, making it more difficult for your heart to pump blood through your system. When you're inflamed, you're also more likely to pack on weight, your energy is low, and your appearance suffers. A recent ten-year study of four thousand middle-aged adults found that just twenty minutes of moderate exercise a day reduced inflammation by at least 12 percent. And this occurred regardless of the BMI or weight of the participants.

The reduction of inflammation may occur due to protein molecules called *cytokines* in the bloodstream, which is released by both your fat and muscle tissues in big doses each time you exercise.

Better Immunity

Unless you're really sick—fever, upset stomach, body aches—moderate exercise (easy walking or jogging with a slightly elevated heart rate) will improve your immunity. So don't allow congestion or a mild head cold to deter you from working out (just don't go all-out, as arduous workouts lasting an hour or more tend to reduce immunity temporarily).

In the longer term, exercise also has a measurable effect on immunity, including one's cancer risk. Research indicates that exercisers have a 40 to 50 percent lower risk of colon cancer, a 30 to 40 percent lower risk of breast cancer (which isn't just good news for the women in your life, as men get breast cancer as well), a 10 to 30 percent lower risk of prostate cancer, and a 20 to 30 percent lower risk of lung cancer than non-exercisers.

Better Hormonal Profile

When you follow the exercise program outlined in this chapter, you'll enjoy a nice hit of testosterone and human growth hormone—it's designed specifically to make this happen. Your adrenals will also give off a beneficial charge, as will supporting hormones like aldosterone (which regulates sodium excretion) and vasopressin, which regulates blood plasma.

To sum it all up: there's barely a system—or a function—in your body that isn't improved by exercise. The body is designed to move and functions best when in motion. *We're supposed to live our lives that way.*

So keep moving, as much as possible. And not just in the gym: more and more research is indicating that movement the other twenty-three hours of each day may contribute just as much to your long-term health.

WAKE UP GREAT

Men and women love the dawn, for its freshness,
For its promise of new beginnings.
In the morning, therefore, I am not frightened
That I have chosen to live a life
Unlike that of other young men.

—ANATOLY IVANESHKI, "THE NON-CONFORMIST"

Your mind is unusually flexible and creative when you first emerge from sleep; testosterone is also at a high, and, if you're a morning person like me, so is your energy, sex drive, and focus.

Whether you managed to get a restful seven-and-a-half hours or tossed and turned all night, what you do in the first thirty to forty-five minutes after you wake up can set the stage for your entire day. So it's essential not to jump into a lot of meaningless, hamster-wheel busywork right when you wake up. As much as you may be tempted to hop online and start responding to email or checking your favorite websites, use those golden minutes deliberately.

Here are my top eight tips for waking up great:

1. Meditate ten minutes before going to bed. See chapter 6 for how to do this. When you don't take a brief transition period before sleep from the busyness and intensity of your day, you often wind up tossing and turning for an hour or more rather than finding your way effortlessly to restfulness and the safety of dreaming. Thoughts, regrets, ideas, and memories from the day past, and anxiety over the day to come, tend to bounce around in your head like pinballs. So this ten to fifteen minutes isn't really another obligation. It will ultimately end up saving you time by clearing your mind of stress. You'll also sleep much better and will wake up with more clarity and ease.

2. Keep a pen and paper next to your bed. I have ideas all the time—as I drift off, in the middle of the night, and when I wake up—and you probably do too. The problem is that when you try to hang on to them, they become another stressor, a niggling item on your to-do list: an item to remember to remember.

At night, there's a simple solution to this: keep a pen and paper by your bed so you can jot those nighttime insights down. Half of them probably won't be worth much—but the other half just might be sheer gold. Regardless, getting them down on paper will clear them from your mental whiteboard—giving you space and time to relax and unwind fully.

3. Meditate fifteen minutes upon waking. This is the best time for meditation: focusing on your breath, being gentle with yourself, listening to your breath. I consider it essential.

4. Expose yourself to natural sunlight. Guys who camp regularly are familiar with the way the body adapts naturally to an early-to-bed, early-to-rise schedule when you're out in the wild. We're hardwired for activity during daylight hours and for rest when it's dark. One of the best ways to tell your nervous system that it's time to get up and at 'em is to get yourself out in the sunshine. Kill two birds with one stone by meditating near a window—or, if weather permits, in the great outdoors. Another option? Sleep with your curtains open so that daylight streams into your room when it's time to wake up.

5. Stay away from email or texting for your first waking hour. Life can wait; it already has for seven hours or so, and another sixty minutes won't make a difference. Assert your autonomy over the many voices clamoring for your attention by insisting that the first hour of your day is all about getting in touch with your needs and how you want your day to unfold.

6. Roll out your feet. The fascia (connective tissue) on the bottoms of your feet is connected to a long band of tissue that runs up the back of your calves, thighs, glutes, and back, and terminates at the base of your skull. At night, this tissue can shorten, making standing (and, of course, walking and running) subtly uncomfortable. Take a minute or two to roll out the bottoms of each foot using a tennis ball or golf ball. And go easy! It should feel good, not painful, as nothing you do at this hour should assault your system.

7. Take a hot shower. You're probably doing this anyway, but showering improves circulation and can facilitate the movement of beneficial, lubricating synovial fluid in your joints and spine. If you have a back that's prone to injury, it's a good idea to take a warm shower prior to exercise if you work out in the morning.

8. Eat something healthy. Here's a healthy smoothie that I drink first thing in the morning. It's fast, delicious, and amazing for you:

> 1 tsp Aiya "Ceremonial" Matcha Green Tea Powder
> 1 serving Vega Sport Vegan Protein Powder (chocolate)
> 1 tsp organic coconut oil (I use Dr. Bronner's fair trade organic)
> 1 tsp MCT Oil (NOW Sports)
> 1 tsp red palm oil
> 1 tbsp organic avocado
> handful of organic blueberries
> sprinkle of turmeric (a little less than ¼ tsp)
> sprinkle of cayenne pepper (a little less than ¼ tsp—careful, it has a bite!)
> ¼ cup rice milk
> 3 cups filtered water

Blend it all up and enjoy!

SLAY THE EXCUSE DRAGON

Okay, so you understand that you should be exercising. And over and over, you start out on a new program brimming with energy and focus, putting in diligent workouts for a couple of weeks, seeing some initial results and feeling great . . . only to come smack up against one or more common motivation-sucking excuses. Happens to the best of us.

The problem is when a single workout missed for a legitimate reason becomes a week, two weeks, or a month of workouts—at which point, you can no longer call yourself a guy who exercises regularly but missed a few workouts—you have to call yourself a nonexerciser who needs to get back into the habit.

I don't want that to happen to anyone reading this. I want Your New Prime exercise program to be the last workout system you ever begin—because you'll never go off it. If you want your second act to really be Your New Prime, exercise simply has to become a real, regular, non-negotiable daily habit. Your family, coworkers, and friends should know that you're an exerciser, and you should enlist them in helping you stick to your program. You may even want to take a few people you care about right along with you on your new fitness crusade—which is a great gift to give to someone.

Excuses wreak havoc on an exercise program because time after time, *consistency* has been shown to be the number one factor that determines the efficacy of an exercise plan. It's not how intensely and diligently you perform a single workout—it's how rigorously you stick to an entire workout program. Three mind-blowing workouts in a month are far less effective in getting you healthy and strong than twenty reasonably good ones in the same time frame.

I've been a regular exerciser for over four decades, and my life is as busy as anyone's. Here are some of the excuses that pop up for me—and some of the ways I've figured out how to get around them.

"I Don't Have Time"

All the time, I hear people say they don't have the time for exercise. What that really means is *exercise isn't a priority for me yet.* How much TV did you watch last week? How much time did you spend on Facebook? How much time watching YouTube videos, or porn, or partying with friends, or doing other time-wasting activities?

I'm not saying don't ever do those things—but if the combined total time you spend on all those activities in a week is more than three hours, then you have time to exercise. If it's more than six hours, you have *plenty* of time.

Let's say you're a corporate warrior who works sixty hours a week. On top of that I'll give you a full ten hours a night to sleep (just to show you don't have to cut down on sleep to fit exercise into your life). Even on that very tight schedule, you still have *thirty-eight hours* in the week during which you can, with a little effort, "find time" to exercise.

Barack Obama is a religious exerciser. So, reportedly, was George W. Bush when he was in office. Whoever you are, whatever the circumstances of your life and family, I can't imagine you have as many pressing issues clamoring for your attention as those guys.

I'll also add that exercise improves your focus, mood, and overall mental health for about twenty-four hours after you work out—meaning that you're more productive and attentive at work or with your family on days when you exercise than on days when you don't. So remember that even if your hour at the gym subtracts an hour from your time at work, it also makes those hours at work all the more productive.

"I'm Embarrassed to Show My Body"

Being embarrassed about one's body is a big one for gym newbies. They think of a health club as a club of superfit, model-and-bodybuilder types, and that if they show themselves, people will wonder who the new out-of-shape guy is.

It doesn't happen. Not in that way, anyway. The fact is that people are way too into themselves (sometimes comically so) to notice a new guy. Gyms are great, but they're narcissistic places. Once you venture inside, you'll also notice a wide variety of fitness levels among the people there—beginners, intermediates, and the very occasional badass, tossing around dumbbells weighted in the triple digits. And as intimidating as they may seem at first, advanced guys were beginners once, too, and they are often very supportive of newer guys and willing to help out if needed.

Personally, when I see new guys (or girls) in the gym, people who clearly have a long journey ahead of them, I'm inspired. It's easy for me to get to the gym; it's been a habit for decades, and I feel quite at home there. But new people have much bigger obstacles to overcome, and a much tougher row to hoe than I do at this point in my life. If you're new to the gym, and new to the process of exercising intensely, know that many people are likely saying little silent cheers for you.

"I Have Joint Pain"

If you have joint pain, join the club, buddy. Whether you're a veteran exerciser or have never darkened a gym door, you probably have a few recurrent aches and pains in your back, knees, shoulders, or elsewhere.

Don't ignore real orthopedic issues. If you have a painful or activity-limiting injury that keeps coming back, get it checked out by a sports med doc or a reputable physical therapist before jumping into a workout program. But aside from that, those little pains, pops, and creaks that most of us have will likely be helped—rather than hurt—by a solid workout program.

Even if you are told to avoid certain activities—low squatting on a stiff knee, for instance—there are so many options, in the gym and out of it, that you're sure to find an activity that doesn't irritate an injury. When I'm in pain, swimming is a zero-impact option that I often turn to for a killer workout.

Concurrently, you can enlist the help of a smart trainer (or, if you have more serious issues, a physical therapist) to give you a specific stretching-and-strengthening program that will address your injuries and help make them better.

For all but the most serious injuries, though, "rest" is an overrated cure-all. Unless something is genuinely broken, most sports medicine doctors recommend light activity, or "active rest," rather than full-on, medically sanctioned lethargy until the pain subsides.

"I Can't Get Motivated"

Lack of motivation is very common at the beginning of an exercise program. You're trying to get into a new, admittedly time-consuming habit, maybe you're sore, maybe you're stressed and tired, and exercise seems like a logical stressor to eliminate from your life.

At first, the solution is, like the saying goes, to *just do it*: get over the hump of resistance, go to the gym (or out on the road), get yourself started, and five minutes in you'll feel great and wonder why you even thought about skipping your workout. You may face the hurdle of having to force yourself to get out there for the first few weeks, but as habit and routine start to form, it becomes much easier to continue.

Long-term lack of motivation, however, may warrant more serious consideration. If you're hating your workouts and dread even the thought of exercise, you may have jumped in too fast and hard (not uncommon for hard chargers!), and your body really needs a break. Alternatively, you may have simply chosen an exercise modality that doesn't agree with you. And though the basic template I recommend in this chapter is the most up-to-date and effective system for developing real-life functional fitness (and there are many options within that template), it's also not the only way to increase your fitness or to get a good workout. You may need to shift gears and commit to something else for a while.

The best motivation comes from the *love* of an activity. According to the fitness expert Frank Forencich, the movement *is* the motivation. If you don't fall in love with the movements I recommend in this chapter (and with how they make you look and feel), find something that does get you excited and motivates you. If you fall out of love with a given modality, shift gears again until you find something your body likes more. Movement should feel good. You should look forward to it. If it doesn't, and you don't, figure out why and make a change.

"Exercise Hurts"

I'll allow that when you commit to a hard run or a tough lift, your muscles may burn a little during exercise, and they may be a little sore for the next couple of days, too. That's part of what you sign up for when you commit to getting stronger, more enduring, and more mobile. Personally, I'm at least a little sore somewhere on my body all the time. I consider it a badge of honor, a mark of being a regular exerciser.

But if exercise *really* hurts—you feel pain in your joints rather than your muscles, or you have debilitating soreness that lasts seventy-two hours or more—you're almost certainly pushing too hard.

Your body is an adaptive machine, capable of becoming much stronger, more flexible, and more enduring—but only when you slowly build up your tolerance for exercise. Rush things, and you'll wind up hurt, especially now that you're out of your teens. So take it slow: you're creating a habit that will hopefully last the rest of your life. If you do overdo it, switch to a lower-intensity activity (ideally one that gently increases circulation in the affected areas) until the intense soreness dissipates, and then get started again—this time using lower weights and lower volume than before.

"Exercise Is Expensive"

Exercise isn't expensive. The idea that you need a $5,000 rowing machine with incrementally stacked weights to exercise your back muscles—when you could hang from a tree branch or a set of monkey bars at your local park, do some rows or pull-ups, and get the same or better results—is a raging falsehood propagated by the fitness industry. Of course the people who own gyms want you to believe that fitness requires massive, expensive machines to get fit: that's how they get people to join the gym and keep coming back.

But I'm here to tell you that you can get a great workout (a better one than you get with machines, in my opinion) in a tiny space using absolutely nothing. Toys are nice to have, but they don't make or break a workout program; your commitment and perseverance does. Convicts in lockdown build and maintain impressive physiques because they're committed to the endeavor, not because they have high-tech exercise gear.

As for truly unavoidable expenses, they're actually fairly minimal. A basic gym membership at a more than adequate commercial gym will set you back about thirty to fifty bucks a month. If you decide to go the trainer route (something you should consider), ask if you can train with a friend and split the cost. Most trainers will be more than happy to accommodate you.

As for apparel, good shoes are about the only semimajor investment. I prefer to go barefoot whenever I do mobility or strength work, but I also have a pair of Vibram FiveFingers shoes, which have individual pockets for each toe, and numerous pairs of minimalist shoes that I use when I run. The only time I wear full-on shoes is when there's a risk of losing my footing (or my toes), such as when I'm pushing a weighted sled.

I recommend you at least consider going barefoot, or using Vibrams or minimalist shoes whenever possible. Connecting with and drawing energy directly from the ground is very energizing and empowering. And though there is some controversy surrounding minimalist shoes,

I strongly believe that the bones of our feet need the impact that barefoot and minimalist training provides to keep them strong. Cushioned shoes rob us of this beneficial impact, and they eventually cause our bones and joints to weaken and become more susceptible to injury.

If you need more support during higher-impact activities, go with the lightest shoes you can comfortably handle, and try to incorporate shoes with less support over time.

With all your other workout attire, feel free to go shabby: old T-shirts, faded sweats, the hoodie from your college days. You don't need to be the well-groomed, perfectly attired metrosexual at the gym who never breaks a sweat. You're not there to be seen; you're there to grunt and sweat and get in touch with your long-buried animal self. Be comfortable looking bad in the gym—so you can look great out of it.

DITCH YOUR CHAIR

The Chumash Indians lived and thrived along the coast of what is now California for almost thirteen thousand years before Europeans descended on them in the 1500s, bringing with them new religious, agricultural, and technological practices. When members of the Chumash were invited to see the interior of a church that Spanish settlers had built, they were baffled by the benches. They didn't know what they were for. What was the point of having benches when you could sit or squat quite comfortably right on the floor, for as long as you wished? In thirteen thousand years of living quite successfully off the resources of the coastline of western North America, the Chumash had never thought to invent a chair.

Perhaps they were on to something.

The innocuous chair—and its derivatives, the recliner, the couch, and the ergonomic car seat—may be among the most dangerous items in your home and office. Whether or not a person exercises regularly, five or more hours a day of sitting is associated with the following head-to-toe problems:

CARDIOVASCULAR

Sit for a long time and your muscles burn less fat than they would otherwise. Blood flow slows down, which allows fat to pool and, potentially, clog the heart. Prolonged sitting is also linked with high blood pressure, high cholesterol, and a higher risk of cardiovascular disease.

BRAIN

Ever notice that when you're stuck on a problem, you often happen on a solution when you stand up to get a snack or visit the bathroom? It's not an illusion. Without your muscles working to pump blood and oxygen through your brain, function slows and you miss out on mood- and brain-enhancing chemicals—resulting in a "foggy" brain. Personally, I get my best ideas when I'm running.

PANCREAS

The pancreas produces insulin, which helps you metabolize sugar. Idle muscles are less sensitive to insulin, so they metabolize sugar less efficiently. When the pancreas senses that your blood sugar is still elevated, it cranks out more insulin. "Insulin sensitivity"—a metric for how well your body clears sugar from your bloodstream—can drop after just one day of prolonged sitting, and it can eventually lead to diabetes.

NECK, BACK, AND SHOULDERS

Repetition of any activity—from assembly line work to jogging to typing on a computer—causes strain in muscles, joints, bones, and connective tissue. Sitting may seem like a passive activity, but in fact it's no different from these other activities, and because we tend to do so much of it, it may be worse. Most of us are slouchers—we round our shoulders forward and allow our heads to drift toward the computer screen. Lots of time in this position results in a constellation of problems in the hips, shoulders, and neck that can cause pain, pinched nerves, and the degeneration of disks.

It's funny that an entire industry has sprung up around "ergonomic" chairs, when it's the chairs themselves that are the problem! The phrase "ergonomic chairs" reminds me of the phrase "healthy cigarette." Even sitting on a ball, which some people swear by, is still sitting.

Got back pain? Sit less.

MUSCLES

You should know this one by now: the less you use your muscles, the smaller, softer, and weaker they get. This is bad news all around. Less muscle means you gain fat more easily, and your mobility—particularly in the hips—suffers. You know that super-flat-butt look that so many older guys develop? That's from sitting. Not a look you want to cultivate.

BONES

Dense, strong bones come from bearing weight. The less you move around—even doing seemingly simple activities like standing and walking—the lighter and weaker your bones become.

The bottom line: sitting sucks. It's antiexercise. It the antithesis of how I want to live my life—I want to live it actively, in motion, in action. Sitting is also an inherently stressed-out position: you're curled up into yourself, like a frightened animal, taking up as little space as possible. As I point out in chapter 1, research has suggested that physical posture has a profound influence on your mood, as well as on levels of testosterone and cortisol.

So you should strive, in our deskbound world, to spend as little time as possible sitting down.

Unrealistic? Perhaps—if you accept the default settings for work and play that most everyone else accepts. Personally, I have a stand-up desk that I use at least half the time I have to do sit-down type work. I know people who swear by treadmill desks, too, which are not as ridiculous as they sound: you amble at a barely detectable one to two miles an hour, but over the course of a week that means that you've walked a good forty-five miles more than you would otherwise, which quickly adds up to some pretty serious mileage—and health benefits. Can you imagine how much weight you might lose if you started walking forty-five miles a week? And you never get the exhausted, too-stiff-to-move feeling that invariably settles in after a long day in a chair. I'm actually standing up right now as I write this chapter!

Other antisitting ideas: move around as much as possible while you watch TV, stand and pace while you talk on the phone (or get a Bluetooth wireless headset), do calisthenics during commercial breaks. When you put in a long day in the office, set a timer to sound every fifteen minutes, and take a sixty-second movement break, whatever else you're doing (I like to crank out twenty pushups every fifteen minutes. Over a day's work in the office, that translates to a pretty decent miniworkout.).

All this movement—known to scientists as non–exercise activity thermogenesis, or NEAT—adds up to better health and fitness. One of your major fitness goals should be to get as much of it as you can in your life.

On top of getting as much NEAT as you can, you'll also want to fold certain antisitting stretches and strengthening moves into your workout program. And guess what? I've included those for you in the workout program at the end of this chapter.

FIT AT FORTY . . . AND BEYOND

Before I set about talking about how to get fit, we should talk about what I mean by *fitness* for a guy over forty.

Sit through an evening of the Olympic games on television and you'll see a vast array of different body types: squat, thick weightlifters; lean, well-muscled sprinters; light, lithe marathoners; all of them at the pinnacle of fitness for their individual events.

So which of them is the fittest?

The answer, of course, is all of them—*for their specific sport.* The marathoner can run at a slow pace for hours, but the weightlifter's warm-up weight would crush him. The weightlifter can toss a refrigerator around with ease, but the marathoner's recovery jog would leave him panting and retching.

We tend to define fitness very narrowly—as the ability to perform a single, specialized task, or simply as the ability to look a certain way with our shirts off.

As an over-forty guy, you need to break out of this narrow view of fitness and start thinking more broadly. Think about fitness not as the ability to run a marathon or rock a pair of board shorts, but primarily as optimal, vital, pain-and-disease-free *health.* Looking good—and performing well athletically—are nice side effects, but at this phase in your life, they aren't the main goals. Before any of that other stuff, you want to be supremely healthy.

If a fitness program makes you sick, causes you pain, or makes you less able to meet the challenges of life, *it's not the right fitness program for you.* You've probably met people who train so fanatically that they're useless outside the gym, out of the pool, or off the road. They leave it all in the gym, and they're exhausted everywhere else.

I think that's foolish. I know hard, passionate training, as I've done it my whole life. But I'm not trying to relive my glory days. It doesn't bother me too much if I'm not as strong or fast or durable as I was in my twenties. Instead of worrying about keeping up with my younger self or breaking the personal performance records I set decades ago, I'm going to make sure what I do in the gym (and on the trail, and in the boxing studio) makes my life outside it better.

When people ask me what I train for, I say "life." I train to be better able to rise to the challenges presented by living right now—may they be physical, mental, or emotional. I'm training not just to perform well and look good, but also to be more resilient and resistant to injury, so that I can stay fully engaged in the game of life as long as possible. The type of physical training I do makes me better able to handle it—not worse.

This sounds like an obvious point, but I see so many guys throwing themselves into specialized exercise programs that essentially cripple them that it's worth mentioning up front. It's a good reminder that if an exercise program ever leaves you feeling constantly run-down and burned-out (brief, not-too-unpleasant soreness is an exception), it's a bad program, and you should back off it or quit altogether.

Fundamentally, the system I present here—and any smart, effective exercise system for a man over forty—will train you like a general-purpose athlete, not a runner, or a cyclist, or a CrossFitter, but as someone who's fit for life first, and all-around athletics second. If there were a decathlon for over-forty men, I would hope that anyone who has been doing the program outlined in this book for a few months would feel good about signing up and giving it a go.

STOP OBSESSING OVER THE SIX

"Get shredded!"

"Lose your gut!"

"See your six-pack in six weeks!"

"Six-minute abs!"

If you're even a casual consumer of fitness magazines, books, DVDs, and the like, these phrases sound all too familiar. Starting in the mid-nineties, the six-pack became the sine qua non of fitness: if you have one, you must be fit; if you don't, you're a tub of lard.

I don't buy it. I happen to be pretty lean—I recently tested at just over 10 percent body fat—and I work out and watch what I eat meticulously. But I also realize that my genetics (in this case, anyway) did me right. I'd probably remain fairly lean (maybe a four-pack in strong overhead light?) even if I curbed way back on my exercise plan.

For other guys, it's a different story: they can diet and work out more diligently than I do for months and never see a single ab. It's just not in the cards for them. For these people, they'd have to diet and exercise so strenuously that even if they finally did unearth their abs, they'd have to lead a 24-7, 365-day life of asceticism and self-denial in order to maintain them. It would literally be a full-time job. Just as it is for professional models and actors—who are paid handsomely, by the way, for their willingness to suffer.

And who wants that?

Reality check: a 2003 study revealed that for men, a healthy body fat percentage is one that's somewhere between 10.8 and 21.7 percent. If you're under 22 percent (almost forty-five pounds of fat at a body weight of two hundred pounds), you're already at a level that science tells us is reasonably healthy, and losing weight won't necessarily make you healthier.

That's not to say you shouldn't try to get leaner; that's also not to say, let's all bulk up to 22 percent body fat. It's just to say that depending on structure, activity level, and genetics, some people can actually carry a substantial amount of body fat and still be exceptionally healthy.

For those of us out there who still harbor dreams of getting—and staying—in the single-digit body fat club, consider the following recent body fat measurements of elite-level male athletes:

- one-hundred- to two-hundred-meter sprinters: 6.5 percent

- marathoners: 6.4 percent

- "weight class" athletes (boxers and wrestlers): 7–8 percent

- body weight–supported sports (canoers/kayakers/swimmers): 13 percent

- off season–physique athletes: 14–15 percent

- contest day–physique athletes: 4–5 percent

Impressive numbers, to be sure. But bear in mind that these athletes are (1) in the prime of their athletic life, (2) on a superintense and rigorous training and dieting schedule, and (3) do not maintain the same level of leanness in the off-season. These athletes look this way only when they are peaking: training their hardest, eating their cleanest, resting their best.

Also note that off-season-physique athletes—and some in-season pro athletes—are actually *not* obsessively, fanatically lean; instead, they maintain a level of body fat that's very sustainable and realistic for most guys.

If, for a brief time, you want to work out and diet single-mindedly, and then snap a picture when the day comes before resuming a more temperate lifestyle, I say go for it. But bear in mind that it's not sustainable—and I sincerely hope that most of us have better things to do.

The eight-by-eight-inch square of flesh on your abdomen does not define who you are as an athlete, a man, or a human being. If you're going to obsess over something in your health and fitness, obsess over feeling better, moving better, and performing better. A six-pack may follow . . . or it may not. Either way, you're healthier and happier for it. And that's a win-win.

THE FITNESS TRIPOD: MOBILITY, STRENGTH, ENDURANCE

There are three major components to my training system, none of which can exist without the other two:

1. Mobility

Mobility is first because it's one that we often ignore, and it's one we over-forty guys tend to lose quickly.

Mobility refers to the ability of each joint to express a full range of motion in a healthy, stable manner. It also refers to your ability to move your entire body through space with control, comfort, and ease—in virtually any direction, at virtually any speed.

If any of these three components of New Prime fitness are equated with exceptional athleticism, it's mobility. Not all great field athletes are super strong or enduring, but the vast majority of them are exceptionally mobile. It's what makes sports exciting to watch. An NFL trainer I know told me that his job is to prevent players from throwing out their backs or straining their hamstrings while tying their shoes. His job, in other words, was to keep them moving well, in all planes of motion—on the field and off it. That's what this part of your program is about, too.

To some guys, mobility may appear unsexy, and they may feel inclined to skip this slower, more meditative part of the workout. Get that idea out of your head. Mobility is not only a key to athleticism, it's also a major key to joint health and longevity. The ability to rise from the floor without using your hands (a rudimentary test of full-body mobility) is a major predictor of longevity. I don't care how long you can jog without stopping—if you can't get off the floor without seven grunts, four groans, and two extended breaks on the way up, you're out of shape and well on the way to becoming the next featured actor in the famous "I've fallen and I can't get up" ads. No one wants to be that guy.

Joint degeneration results from *repetitive use*. This comes from continually moving your joints in the same way, over and over again, along the same limited range of motion that everyday, modern life demands of you. That's why you creak when you stand up from the floor: your hips, lower back, and shoulders aren't used to even that mildly challenging amount of movement anymore. Mobility work restores those more extreme ranges of motion so that pain-free athletic movement becomes possible again.

This is why you shouldn't skip your mobility work.

Every New Prime workout begins with a mobility sequence that, once you get the hang of it, will take you ten minutes or less. It will address most of the common mobility problems that desk-bound guys our age tend to encounter: tight hips, rounded shoulders, tight calves, "stuck" rib cage, and poor rotation in the upper spine. You'll start most mobility workouts with five minutes of foam rolling (manipulating muscle and connective tissue by rolling your body over a cylindrical piece of stiff Styrofoam), and then you'll move on to a series of movements intended to increase the pain-free range of motion in your major joints.

There are literally thousands of different mobility drills out there. (If you have a day or two to spare, do a search for "mobility exercises" on YouTube. You may never return.) And over time, your repertoire of these moves will gradually expand, as trainers, friends, and other sources introduce you to new moves that you like. That's fine. But the mobility sequence in Your New Prime workout program is foundational to moving well and addressing our most common mobility issues. Try the mobility warm-up once and you'll notice an immediate difference in how you stand, breathe, and feel. Do it five to seven times a week for thirty days and you'll feel like a new man.

2. Strength

Strength refers to a muscle's ability to contract under some kind of load. The heavier the load, the stronger the muscle.

Muscle tissue exists in two broad categories: (1) type I muscle fibers, which are red, and are typically smaller and more enduring; and (2) type II muscle fibers, which are white, and are typically bigger and stronger.

How much of each type of muscle fiber exists in each of your muscle groups is an individual matter (the guy you know with shoulder muscles like overripe cantaloupes probably has deltoids packed with type II fibers), and it can help determine which sports and activities you do well in.

As I've mentioned, guys tend to lose some muscle as we age, but if you don't exercise, much of that muscle loss comes from your store of type II muscle fibers; it's why you don't see too many eighty-year-olds bounding up stairs like ten-year-old boys. But if we take steps to stem the tide of type II muscle loss—by using some heavier weights and faster movements when we exercise—we can hold on to our ability to express strength and, when necessary, move quickly and powerfully. Your New Prime workout program includes exercises that will stimulate both types of muscle fibers.

Strength also refers to your ability to coordinate action in any number of the six hundred muscles in your body. A lunge exercise, for example, requires coordinated action in the muscles that surround the spine, hips, knees, ankles, and core. If any one of these areas fails, you won't be able to complete the lunge.

So strength, in this program, isn't just about having muscle—it's also about being able to use it well. I like to think of strength as a skill that involves not just muscle, but also your brain, spinal column, and nervous system as well. So even though some of these workouts won't necessarily make your muscles sore, know that your body is still learning—getting better, and therefore stronger—from head to toe.

3. Endurance

Endurance is your ability to perform physical work for an extended period. Your muscles are involved in endurance activities, of course (since you're moving through space), but the primary limiter of your ability to perform endurance activities is your cardiovascular system: heart, lungs, and peripheral circulatory system.

Long-distance running, of course, is considered an endurance activity; so are cycling and swimming, and anything you do on a cardio machine at the gym.

I'm going to argue, however, that it's much better for you (not to mention less time-consuming) to build endurance and cardiovascular health *not* through a lot of relatively slow, plodding "cardio" activities, such as you see people doing in the gym. I don't have a problem with jogging or cycling as fun activities to do *in addition* to your regular workouts (I like a good mountain bike ride through nature as much as the next guy), but to build and improve endurance, I suggest you use **P**eak **R**epetition **I**ntervals with **M**aximum **E**ffort, or PRIME Workouts.

PRIME Workouts are pretty simple in execution: instead of lacing up your sneakers and jogging, rowing, or elliptical-ing at a steady pace for forty minutes or more, you warm up thoroughly (using the mobility exercises in this chapter), choose two to three challenging, full-body exercises, arrange them in a circuit, and then go at a hard pace for a very short period on each movement—say, thirty seconds. Between exercises, you rest for a designated period, say, two minutes. Then you repeat the work-rest cycle on these same moves for a set number of repetitions through the circuit—say, three.

Then you go home.

A little math will show you that that entire workout, excluding your warm-up, will last at most thirty minutes, and if you've never done this style of training before, you'll probably think I'm going easy on you because I don't think you can handle a real workout.

I implore you to try one of these workouts before you judge it and get back to me on that. PRIME Workouts are admittedly brief—that's one of their many virtues—but they're also very taxing. Assuming you follow the directions and push yourself hard in those work periods, your heart rate will skyrocket during—and between—those thirty-second bouts of effort. All the vessels along your entire circulatory system will dilate to accommodate the tidal wave of oxygenated blood that your working muscles will be demanding. The first time or two you try it, you may feel a little light-headed (when was the last time you ran anywhere as fast as you could?), but pretty soon you'll find that PRIME Workouts feel amazing. Your limbs tingle with life. Your breath feels clear, expansive. Your thoughts will even feel clearer. Hormonally, PRIME Workouts are also a winner, as adrenaline and testosterone course through you, making you feel like you could conquer the world.

I'll also add that PRIME Workouts build and maintain muscle mass far more effectively than slow cardio, which, some studies have indicated, can actually cause muscle loss. It also works all three of the body's energy systems—aerobic, glycolytic, and ATP-PC—each of which runs on a different type of fuel but which work in tandem to power up different levels of effort and intensity in the body. Straight-up aerobic training focuses primarily on just one of these engines.

As I've designed them, PRIME Workouts are flexible, too, so you can perform them on a track, stationary bike, rowing machine, hill—even in a gym using body weight–exercises like squats, burpees, and push-ups (as long as you do them *fast*). You can choose your work interval, your rest interval, and the number of repetitions you perform, based on your fitness level and your goals. You're therefore less likely to injure yourself doing my PRIME Workouts than you are by doing long, slow cardio or by repeating the same high-intensity workouts over and over again.

It's also—if you haven't gathered this already—a hell of a lot of fun.

Can you tell I'm a PRIME fan?

I'll go more into the how-tos of my custom-built PRIME Workouts in a bit. For now, though, understand that this type of training should be a major cornerstone of your workout program—now and forever. This shouldn't be a problem, since you can do these workouts virtually anywhere, anytime, in very little time. And if they sound too challenging for you, fear not—you can always work at your own level, a level that will very quickly rise as your overall fitness improves.

Mobility, strength, endurance—those are the legs of Your New Prime fitness tripod, none of which can stand without the others. Though they're distinct qualities, they're also closely related: your heart won't pound unless your muscles are working, and your muscles won't move well unless you've mobilized them. The mobility workout may make your muscles burn, and your strength workout may make your heart pound. So although each piece of Your New Prime workout program is designed to build one of these specific qualities, there's nonetheless a lot of crossover as well.

That's all by design. The point of this exercise program isn't to chop your body up into separate pieces, or even separate functions, and then build some up while whittling others down (though your body will unquestionably look better on this program!). The point is to improve everything at once, to make your body work better as a whole so you can handle whatever challenges life throws at you.

You'll also be able to handle any athletic challenge you decide to undertake. If, a few months into this program, you decide you want to train for a sprint-distance triathlon, you'll be able to get in shape for it in a matter of a few weeks—not months. If you want to do a mud run with some friends (very fun, by the way), same deal: sign up, specialize your training for a few weeks, and you're literally off to the races. Feel like joining a tennis or racquetball club, or hiking a mountain, or taking a ski weekend? Assuming your joints are healthy and you have the skills, it's all quite doable. The limitation on your ability to do these things won't be poor fitness anymore. In fact, you'll never have poor fitness as an excuse to avoid doing anything from now on. You'll always be game-ready.

A body that's strong, functional, highly adaptable, feels great—and, incidentally, looks pretty awesome too—is attainable for any reasonably healthy guy over forty. This program will put you on a path to getting there.

HOW NOT TO GET FIT: RUNNING MARATHONS

Legend has it that around about 490 BC, a Greek messenger ran the twenty-six-and-change-mile route from Marathon to Athens to announce the Greeks' victory at the Battle of Marathon. Now, a couple of millennia later, about half a million people annually pay hefty entrance fees and spend months preparing to run 26.2 miles in marathons the world over.

I don't necessarily fault them; I've run marathons myself, along with a few other ultra-long-distance running events.

But here's the part of the marathon-origin story that most long-distance runners forget: after he delivered his message, the messenger *died*.

If only he'd had Skype.

And this fleet-footed Greek was a professional messenger. He routinely did runs of this distance. On the day he did his Marathon run, he had *fought* in the Battle of Marathon. Talk about an overachiever.

The same unfortunate fate befell Micah True, the long-distance runner who is one of the heroes of Christopher McDougall's book *Born to Run*. After decades of running distances of up to one hundred miles at a stretch, he died at age fifty-eight while on a routine training run.

It's unlikely you'll suffer the Greek messenger's fate if you decide to run a single marathon and you prepare well for it. But, whatever your buddy at the office, or your Facebook friend Pat, or your son tells you, by no means should you consider long-distance running a viable way to improve your health and longevity, nor should you consider it something to do on a regular basis.

If you are a 120-pound, 8 percent body fat, Nike-sponsored slip of a thing who is obviously genetically suited for such madness (and making good money off it), knock yourself out; it's your livelihood, and you do what you have to do. Failing that, though, running marathons—or even running long distances frequently—is not an effective way to get fit. It may even be bad for your health.

Here's why: As guys, we're highly susceptible to the "more is better" myth. If running two miles three times a week is good for you, we assume that ten miles seven times a week must be *great* for you. It's not so. For one thing, the nutritional requirements of training for and completing a marathon—bars, gels, sports drinks, and the like, all of which are variations on straight sugar—are antithetical to good eating habits. A few long-distance athletes, such as Ironman Dave Scott and ultramarathoner Scott Jurek, eat plant-based diets, so it can be done without eating all the processed, sugary crap. But junk is so ubiquitous at these events, and so much a part of the culture of training, that it can be hard to avoid.

But the ill effects of long-distance running go well beyond its sugar-saturated training culture. According to the cardiologist James O'Keefe, after sixty minutes of strenuous exercise, the heart becomes inflamed. Many marathoners exhibit elevated levels of troponin following a race—an indication that smooth muscle tissue in the heart is literally dying off. Studies have indicated that regular marathoners have 62 percent *more* plaque in their arteries than men of comparable age and risk factors who aren't long-distance runners. They also exhibit scarring in the left ventricle—the chamber of the heart responsible for sending oxygenated blood into the body.

These are scary findings, and they confirm what nonrunners have long been thinking: *all that running can't be good for you.*

To be clear, *all* running isn't bad for you. *Obsessive* running is. When you train for a marathon, you're basically revving your cardiovascular engine into the red zone. The health benefits of running peak when you run a relatively modest ten to fifteen miles a week, for one to two-and-a-half hours, two or three times a week, at a moderate pace. Too much, too fast, too often? You might as well stay on the couch.

Training for a marathon takes a lot of dedication, grit, and determination, and also a willingness to endure physical pain. Those are all commendable attributes on the exercise front, and I applaud your hard work. If you're looking for a way to improve your health and fitness, however, your time and energy is better spent on some of the other activities I recommend in this chapter.

Want to run a marathon so you can cross it off your bucket list, as I did? Go for it. Once. You'll peak for that *one single day* when you're capable of making that run. A few years ago I was signed up for the New York City Marathon, which was then cancelled after Hurricane Sandy. Two weeks later there was another marathon in Santa Barbara that I could have run—but I chose not to, because I'd engineered my training to peak for the exact day of the New York City Marathon, not a day before or after. I didn't feel ready for the Santa Barbara race. Even when you do it right, marathon training is a highly specialized—and artificial—endeavor. It's no way to run your life.

Whatever you do, *don't* train for a marathon to get in shape. Get in shape, and then train for one single marathon. And once you've done it . . . put it behind you.

Love running, and want an easier, faster, more sustainable, and more fun way to get fit? Start running 5Ks (more on that at the end of this chapter).

THE PROGRAM: WHERE TO BEGIN

Okay, this is where the rubber (finally) meets the road.

It's day one, you're psyched, and you're equipped with the best shoes and the crappiest set of sweats you can find. You're ready.

How to begin?

First, you'll need to figure out your starting point. This is essential. You don't start building a house with the chimney, and you don't embark on a journey without knowing your present coordinates. Here's how to locate yourself:

Beginner

Beginners, naturally enough, have either never exercised regularly, or, if they have, they haven't done so consistently (three days a week minimum) for the last three months. By *exercised*, I mean working up a sweat and *deliberately* getting some serious huffing and puffing going (wrestling the occasional grocery bag or wheeling the garbage to the curb doesn't count!). If your doctor has told you that you need to start working out, even if you have been "trying to lately," sorry, buddy, you're still a beginner.

Don't be ashamed to start here, though. The mobility and endurance workouts you'll do will be virtually the same as those of the more advanced exercisers, and the strength workouts you'll do are still very tough. The focus, however, will be on building joint integrity, balance, stability, and control. You won't use big weights on your strength workouts—most of the time you'll be using your body weight only. But these workouts will iron out the kinks in your system, aid in injury prevention and reduction, and prepare your body for working with heavier weights.

Exerciser

If you've been working out regularly for three to six months and have started to feel and notice physical changes (better wind, strength, energy) but haven't come close to maxing out in any of them, you're an "exerciser"—an intermediate-range gym-goer.

This is a great phase to be in.

If you're wavering over whether to call yourself an exerciser or an athlete, choose exerciser. The workouts at the athlete level may or may not be right for you, and you'll still get plenty of challenge—enough to keep you working hard, even for years to come—out of the exerciser-level workouts.

The exerciser strength workouts are all about building strength and muscle; you'll use more conventional exercises with heavier weights for fewer repetitions. This is the level at which you'll start to see and feel many of the changes that this exercise program delivers: less fat, more muscle, better performance.

Athlete

Athlete is an optional phase that I'm including because some guys over forty want an überdifficult level of challenge now and then. They want workouts that would challenge their younger, fitter, more explosive selves; and they want to see how lean, strong, and athletic their New Prime bodies are capable of becoming. If that's you, this is your level.

Unless you have been strength-training, sprinting, and working on mobility religiously for at least six months, *don't jump into this phase*. Give yourself a month in the exerciser level first.

You've been warned.

People who wish to delve into the athlete workouts will find that the exercises are fast-paced and intense at times, slow and intense at others, and always exhausting. When you strength-train, you'll work with weights that approach your maximum; when you do athletic moves (also built in to this level), you'll do so at maximum speed—the idea being to push your body to its limit and elicit as much change from your nervous and muscular systems as possible.

Once you've determined your level, you should spend the first thirty days of your exercise program there.

A WEEK IN YOUR NEW PRIME WORKOUT PROGRAM

Whether you're a beginner, an exerciser, or an athlete, your weekly workout schedule will look more or less like this:

Sunday	Monday	Tuesday	Wednesday	Thursday	Friday	Saturday
Active rest	Mobility program	Mobility program	Mobility program	Fun activity, ideally outdoors	Mobility program	Mobility program
	Strength workout A	PRIME Workout	Strength workout B		Strength workout A	PRIME Workout

The following week will look much the same except that you'll do Strength Workout B twice (on Monday and Friday) and Strength Workout A just once (on Wednesday). Week three will look the same as week one (with A on Monday and Friday, B on Wednesday) and week four will look the same as week two (with the opposite schedule).

Right now, I realize this table doesn't make much sense to you. I hear you asking, *What are Strength Workouts A and B? What are the PRIME Workouts?* We'll get to all that.

For now, just register that:

(1) You'll be doing *three* strength workouts on *nonconsecutive* days during the week. In my example, I use the standard Monday, Wednesday, Friday format, but you can also use Tuesday, Thursday, Saturday, or any other version of that you want. It can vary week to week if you wish; you just need to get all three in each week, alternating workouts A and B each time you do a strength workout.

(2) You'll be doing *two* PRIME (peak repetition intervals with maximum effort) workouts a week on separate *nonconsecutive* days during the week. Once you've slotted in your strength workouts, put your PRIME Workouts in on *separate* days. Don't do a PRIME Workout and a strength workout on the same day.

(3) All strength and PRIME Workouts are preceded by *mobility* workouts. You can do them at other times too, but you must always do them before these workouts. This is nonnegotiable.

(4) One day a week is reserved for a fun, *intense* activity. This could be a challenging hike, an afternoon of Ultimate Frisbee, a 5K race, a mud run, a mountain bike ride, or any team or individual sport that gets your heart rate going (golf doesn't count, Sunday duffer!). Anything fun, active, and *strenuous* counts. Be creative and, ideally, inclusive: this is a good day to spend some time with other athletically minded guys (a little competition is a huge motivator for most of us). Bonus points if the activity is outside.

(5) One day a week is for fun, *relaxing* activity. This is your "active rest" day. Some paddleboarding or surfing, an easier hike or bike ride. Again, think outdoors and social, but this time, take it a little easier. Enjoy the elements. Sure, sweat a little—but save your hard, high-intensity efforts for other days of the week.

Nominally, that makes a seven-day-a-week schedule, but "active rest" is something you should be getting plenty of anyway. It speeds recovery and keeps you from being a total slouchy mess on that free day during the week. I'm just giving you a gentle nudge to remember to do that.

That's the basic structure that beginners, exercisers, and athletes will all follow. The main difference between the three levels will be in your strength workouts—which we will get to shortly.

Within this structure, however, feel free to play around: maybe you need to schedule everything around the fact that you play basketball on Wednesday nights and want to feel fresh for those games. If that's the case, call that your "fun, intense activity," make Tuesday your active rest day (the easiest day of the week), do your strength workouts on Monday, Thursday, and Saturday, and do a PRIME Workout on Friday and Sunday. There are plenty of options.

The primary scheduling strategy is to get your three strength workouts slotted in on nonconsecutive days around other preexisting activities and obligations, and go from there.

Okay, those are the broad strokes of your schedule. Now what exactly do you do in each of those baffling-sounding workouts? Glad you asked. . . .

THE MOBILITY PROGRAM

Sunday	Monday	Tuesday	Wednesday	Thursday	Friday	Saturday
Active rest	**Mobility program**	**Mobility program**	**Mobility program**	Fun activity, ideally outdoors	**Mobility program**	**Mobility program**
	Strength workout A	PRIME Workout	Strength workout B		Strength workout A	PRIME Workout

The first thing you'll do in Your New Prime workouts—regardless of whether you're a beginner, an exerciser, or an athlete—is something that hurts so good.

If you've never gotten friendly with a foam roller—a piece of industrial Styrofoam six inches in diameter and three feet in length—prepare for a few good winces: when you use the roller, your entire body weight will press down on tender, tight spots in your muscles and connective tissue—the same areas that make you whimper when your massage therapist (or well-meaning life partner) digs into them.

But the worse foam rolling hurts, the more you probably need it.

There are conflicting opinions about how and why foam rolling works. Some trainers believe it affects tissue quality by breaking up knots and scarring in your tendons and muscles; others believe it works largely through forcibly relaxing the muscles via the nervous system. My view is that *it doesn't matter*. Foam rolling works. Five or ten minutes of rolling out your major muscle groups will fundamentally affect the way you move and feel—especially if you've never done it before.

I recommend you roll out all your major muscle groups before doing *anything* else in every workout. A good rule of thumb is that you should do one full five-to-ten-minute foam-rolling routine a week for every decade you've been alive. You'll unkink the muscles while turning inward and focusing on breath and sensation as you move.

A high-quality, dense foam roller (the gray or black kind—not the white kind!) costs less than forty bucks, so I highly recommend picking one up, keeping it at home, and rolling out whenever the mood strikes (maybe instead of collapsing on the couch while watching TV). If you've reached forty years old, regardless of whether you've spent more of those years on a bike or on the couch, it's safe to say that your tissue quality is in need of some pretty serious help.

It's almost something you can't do too often. I've indicated time suggestions for each area below for guidance, but if you need more time in any particular area (and you'll know it if you do!), feel free to take it.

Better Movement in Eight Minutes: Foam Rolling

YOUR NEW PRIME FOAM ROLLING PROGRAM AT A GLANCE

Exercise	Duration		Exercise	Duration
Quadriceps	60 seconds		Glutes	30 seconds/side
Adductors	30 seconds/side		Lats	30 seconds/side
IT Band	30 seconds/side		Pecs	30 seconds/side
Calves	30 seconds/side		Upper Back	30 seconds

Quadriceps

Lie facedown on top of the roller, placing it at hip height, perpendicular to your spine. Slowly roll yourself forward, breathing deeply and allowing the roller to sink into muscles along the fronts of your thighs. Adjust the angle of your feet (turning toes inward or outward) each time you roll forward or back. *One minute.*

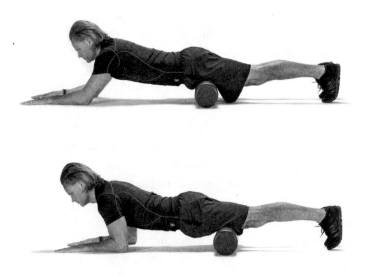

Adductors

Lie facedown with your right hip lifted and your right knee pointed ninety degrees out to the right. Place the roller beneath your right knee, parallel to your spine. Slowly roll along the inside of your right thigh, all the way into the groin. *Thirty seconds per side.*

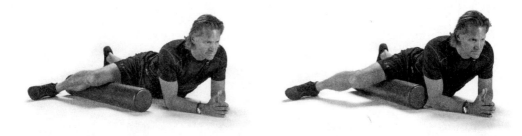

IT Bands

Turn onto your right side, positioning yourself so that the protrusion at the top of your right thighbone is on the roller. Slowly roll along the outside of your right thigh, all the way to your knee. *Thirty seconds per side.*

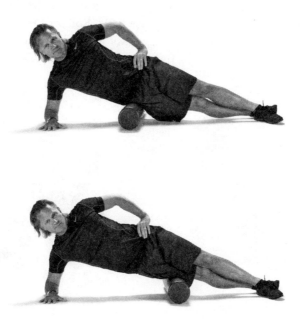

Calves

Sit on the floor with the roller in front of you and place your right foot on top of it. Cross your left leg over your right, allowing your right foot, ankle, and calf to relax completely. Slowly roll along the entire back side of your right calf, all the way up to your knee. Adjust the angle of your right foot (turning toes inside or out) each time you roll forward or back. *Thirty seconds per side.*

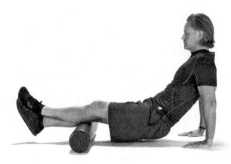 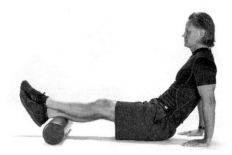

Glutes

Sit on top of the foam roller with your right ankle resting on your left knee. Shift to the right so that most of your weight is on your right sitting bone. Roll forward and back, working the area from the top of your glute muscles, near the lower back, to the lowermost part of the glutes, where they attach to your hamstrings. The entire movement is not more than a few inches. *Thirty seconds per side.*

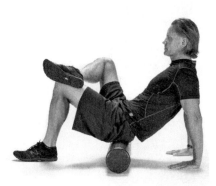 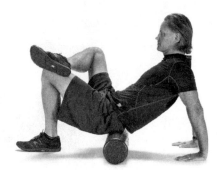

Lats

Lie on your right side, right arm extended overhead, with the roller placed beneath your right armpit. Slowly roll along the right side of your torso, toward the bottom of your rib cage, and back again. *Thirty seconds per side.*

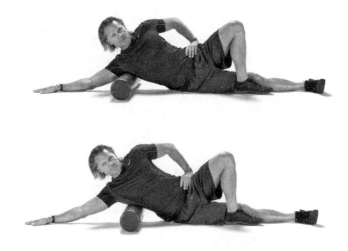

Pecs

Lie facedown on top of a foam roller placed just below your armpits. Extend one arm forward. Press your chest into the foam roller and roll back and forth in small movements. Extend your other arm and repeat. *Thirty seconds per side.*

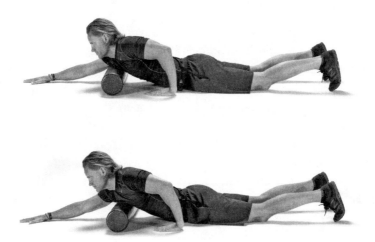

Upper Back

Lie on your back with the roller at shoulder-blade height, perpendicular to your spine. Hug your upper body with your arms, and slowly roll yourself forward and back along the back of your upper rib cage. *Thirty seconds.*

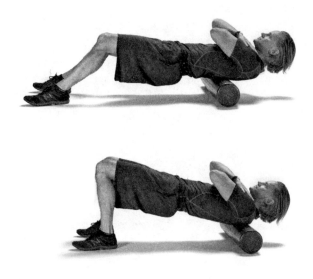

For demos of these exercises, see www.thenewprime.com/primetraining.

Your New Prime Mobility Moves

After foam-rolling, your next item of business in your mobility program is to start moving actively. Many exercise professionals recommend five minutes on a bike or treadmill for this purpose. I disagree. Targeted mobility drills will raise your heart rate and increase joint lubrication and core temperature, while undoing many of the faulty movement patterns—rolled-in shoulders, tight hips, inactive glutes, tight ankles—that we develop from years of sitting on our individual butts. These moves will stretch the muscles in the front of your body while strengthening those in the back—allowing you to move in a way that more closely resembles how our bodies evolved to move.

My good friend Dr. Eric Goodman, a chiropractor, a consultant to elite athletes and celebrities, and the author of the book *Foundation*, argues persuasively that our modern-day lifestyle essentially turns the muscles on the backs of our bodies to mush—and that one major key to long-term postural health and performance is to activate and strengthen the "posterior chain" muscles (glutes, hamstrings, lower back). I agree—and that's why those areas are so much a focus of the mobility program I outline below. (It's also why I appropriated one of the moves from the posture-improving program he pioneered—the "Founder"—to be part of this program. Thanks, Eric!)

As with the foam-rolling drills, there is no reason you should limit your mobility work to before your workouts. Crank out some moves in between meetings at work, or when you need a break from your chair (often), or while waiting for a connecting flight at the airport. These moves are ideal for five-minute, no-sweat movement snacks. And they feel fantastic.

MOBILITY AT A GLANCE

Exercise	Reps/Distance/Time
Hip Flexor Stretch with Overhead Reach	10 seconds in each position
Lying Glute Bridge	10 reps, 3-second hold each
Squat to Stand with Overhead Reach	10 reps
New Prime "Founder" Variation	1–2 slow reps, 15–30-second hold in "Founder" position
Scapular/T-Style Push-Up	5 reps/side
Standing Alternating Quad Stretch	10 reps/side
Forward Inchworm	10 reps
Single-Leg Dead Lift Walk	10 reps/side
Bear Crawl	20 yards
Side Shuffle	20 yards
Carioca	20 yards

For demos of these exercises, see www.thenewprime.com/primetraining.

Hip Flexor Stretch with Overhead Reach

- Assume a half-kneeling position, right knee on the floor, left foot standing in front of you.
- Keeping your torso upright, lunge forward until you feel a stretch in the front of your right hip.
- Maintaining this stretched position, reach your right hand upward.
- Hold for ten seconds, then side-bend to the left.
- Hold for ten seconds, then rotate to the left.
- Hold for ten seconds, then repeat the entire sequence with your right foot forward.

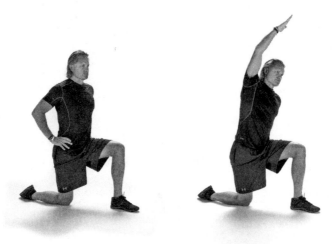

Lying Glute Bridge

- Lie on your back with your knees bent and feet flat on the floor, shoulder-width apart.
- Push down through your feet, lifting your pelvis as high in the air as possible.
- Squeeze your glute muscles for a slow three-count.

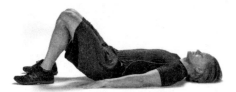 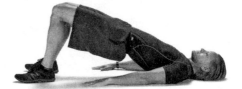

Squat to Stand with Overhead Reach

- Stand with your feet slightly wider than shoulder-width apart, toes pointed slightly outward.
- Bend forward at the hip joints, reaching down toward your feet, ankles, or shins, depending on your flexibility.
- Keeping your feet flat on the floor, drop your hips as low as possible toward the floor while simultaneously straightening your back and lifting your chest high.
- Raise both hands overhead as high as possible, thumbs pointed back behind you.
- Keeping your arms overhead, stand upright.

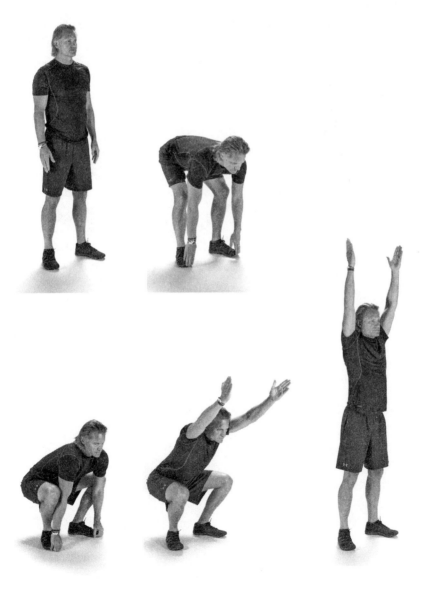

New Prime "Founder" Variation

- Stand about two feet behind a chair, table, or exercise step that's about belly-button high.
- Take three to five deep breaths into your chest, simultaneously lengthening the front of your rib cage and pulling your stomach in as much as possible.
- Keeping your lower back in its natural arch, bend your knees very slightly and place your hands on the implement.
- Keeping your torso long, hinge forward at the hips, pressing your chest toward the floor as much as possible and sliding your hands forward on your prop as you descend.
- Hold the stretched position for fifteen to thirty seconds.
- Remaining bent forward at the hips, slowly bring your arms to your sides with your palms facing outward, thumbs up, and squeeze your shoulder blades together as much as possible.
- Hinging at the hip joints (not the lower back), slowly return to the starting position.

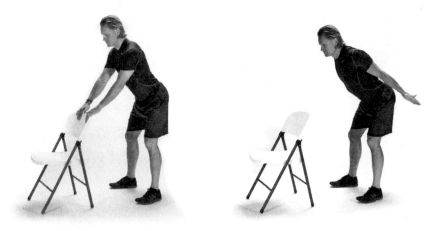

Scapular/T-Style Push-Up

- Assume a push-up position, hands beneath your shoulders, body straight from the crown of your head to your heels.
- Step your left foot forward and place it as close to the outside of your left hand as possible.
- Reach your left hand upward toward the ceiling, rotating back as far as you can.
- Place your left hand back on the floor and step your left foot backward so you are again in push-up position.
- Keeping your body straight, and your shoulders away from your ears, squeeze your shoulder blades together briefly, then return to the neutral push-up position.
- Repeat the movement on your right side, and alternate for the appropriate number of repetitions.

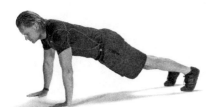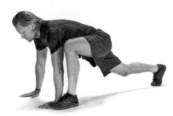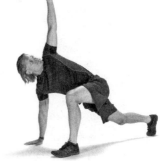

Standing Alternating Quad Stretch

- Assume an athletic stance, feet parallel and shoulder-width apart.
- Step your right foot about six inches to your right, and bend your left leg up behind you, taking hold of your left ankle with your left hand.
- Gently pull your heel toward your butt and hold for a quick one-count.
- Release your left ankle, step your foot back to the ground, and repeat on your opposite side, alternating sides for the appropriate number of repetitions.

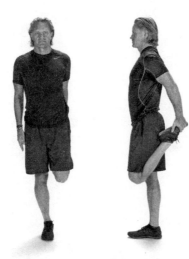

Forward Inchworm

- Assume a push-up position, hands beneath your shoulders, body straight from the crown of your head to your heels.
- Keeping your knees straight and your hands on the floor, walk your feet forward as far as you can.
- Walk your hands forward until you are in pushup position again.

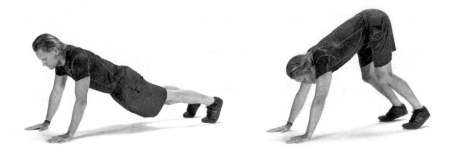

Single-Leg Dead Lift Walk

- Assume an athletic posture, feet parallel and shoulder-width apart.
- Step your right foot forward one normal stride length.
- Keeping your right leg slightly bent, your hips and shoulders square to the floor, and your lower back in its natural arch, hinge forward at the hip joints, extending your left leg up and behind you until your torso and left leg form a straight line, parallel to the floor.
- Lower your left leg and come back to the standing position.
- Repeat the movement, stepping forward with your left leg, and continue the movement, alternating legs for the appropriate number of repetitions.

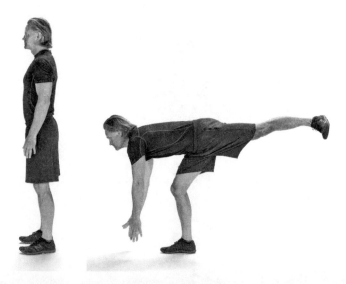

Bear Crawl

- Assume an all-fours position with your knees directly under your hips and your hands directly under your shoulders.
- Flex your ankles forward so that the balls of your feet are on the floor, and lift both knees off the floor.
- Keeping your spine parallel to the floor, slowly raise your right hand and your left foot off the floor and step them forward about six inches.
- Shift your weight onto your right hand and left foot, and repeat the movement on the other side, stepping your left hand and right foot forward.
- Repeat the movement, taking care to lift and lower the hand and opposite foot at the same instant as you travel forward.

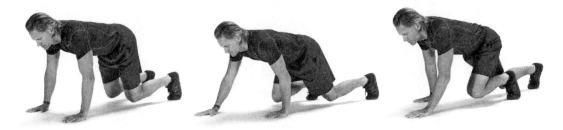

Side Shuffle

- Stand facing forward with your feet parallel and shoulder-width apart.
- Keeping your feet parallel and your eyes and torso aimed directly forward, step your right foot about twelve inches to your right.
- Step your left foot twelve inches to the right.
- Quickly repeat the process, shuffling to the right about twenty yards.
- Change directions, shuffling back to the starting point.

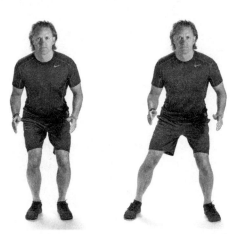

Carioca

- Stand facing forward with your feet parallel and shoulder-width apart.
- Step your left foot in front and to the right of your right foot.
- Step your right foot to the right so your feet are shoulder-width apart again.
- Step your left foot behind and to the right of your right foot.
- Step your right foot to the right so your feet are shoulder-width apart again.
- Quickly repeat the process, alternately stepping in front of and then behind your right foot with your left until you've traveled about twenty yards.
- Change directions, performing the drill back to the starting position.

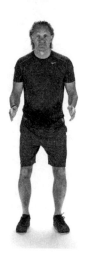 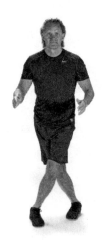 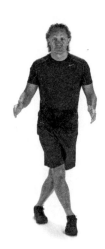

BUILDING STRENGTH

Sunday	Monday	Tuesday	Wednesday	Thursday	Friday	Saturday
Active rest	Mobility program	Mobility program	Mobility program	Fun activity, ideally outdoors	Mobility program	Mobility program
	Strength workout A	PRIME Workout	**Strength workout B**		**Strength workout A**	PRIME Workout

So you've foam-rolled yourself silly and mobilized your joints like a contortionist. Once you get through those warm-up moves, you should be about fifteen minutes in to your workout. Now is when it really gets serious.

GET LOOSE WITH IT

This chapter is all about getting *systematic* with your workout program so you can make measurable, visible progress toward your fitness goals. Over time, however, I want you to discover the glories of spontaneous, random workouts—the kind that just pop up without warning.

Let's say you decide to go to the beach for an afternoon. Some pals and their wives come along, and maybe some of their kids, too. At some point, someone will pull out a Frisbee or a football or some bodyboards, and you'll have a great opportunity to squeeze in a spontaneous little workout that's as low-key or as intense as you want it to be.

Equally, you might live somewhere cold, and have guests in town, and decide to go skating, cross-country skiing, or downhill skiing for an afternoon. It's another chance to steal a workout, sandwiching it between other obligations.

I'm all about being physical as often, and in as many different ways, as I can, and I encourage you—once you've developed a solid fitness foundation—to do the same. At this point, it's the weather, almost more than any other factor, that determines what I'll do on a given day. Do the workouts in this book so you can be ready and eager to pounce on an opportunity to do a new kind of workout or participate in a new type of sport whenever you can.

Unlike the mobility and foam-rolling workouts, the strength workout—which you'll do three times a week, on nonconsecutive days—differs based on your experience level and goals. So this portion of your workout will be different depending on whether you're a beginner, an exerciser, or an athlete. At every level, though, each strength workout consists of at least one movement from each of the following categories:

- upper-body pushing
- lower-body pushing
- upper-body pulling
- lower-body pulling
- core

These five categories cover all the basic movements of the human body, and, combined, will hit all the muscles in your upper, middle, and lower body.

There are gym-goers who like to spend all day working their biceps, or training their forearms or traps or calves. They'll do an hour or more of curl variations, spending several minutes between sets, chatting with friends and flexing in the mirror. These well-meaning gym denizens may try to tell you that you need to follow suit, and that five or six exercises per workout to cover the whole body just ain't enough, bro.

Don't listen to them. For one thing, the "divide and conquer" system, while it may work well for jobless teens with nothing better to do than kill two hours a day in the gym trying to get "huge," won't work for you. You don't have time for it.

It's also not particularly good for you. Sure, some guys who work out that way have huge muscles to show for it (many of whom, it must be said, would be huge regardless of the type of workout they did). But most of the biggest guys you see in the gym also have terrible posture, awful mobility, and a host of latent injuries to show for all that pressing and curling.

Finally, "split system" strength training isn't in line with your goals. Working the whole body at once and using exercises that work many muscle groups at the same time is time-efficient, effective, and, if you commit to it, exhausting. You won't want to do any more than the amount I'm suggesting. And if you want a body that feels great, performs great, *and* looks great, this is the way to go.

These are the types of workouts that old-time strongmen used to do before there were drugs, souped-up supplements, and other elixirs that allowed them to train longer, harder, and more often than normal humans.

The nine tables that follow show the A and B workouts for each experience level (beginner, exerciser, and athlete). On each one you'll see every *exercise* in the workout listed alongside its *movement type* ("upper-body push," or "core," for example), the *reps* (number of times you perform each movement), *sets* (number of times you repeat that same number of repetitions, with rest between sets), and *rest* (the approximate amount of time you take between sets). Find your page, make a copy, and take it with you every time you go to the gym.

On page 144, you will also find an *empty* table that you can copy and use to record your progress on each workout. Run off three copies of that page so you can record your progress on each different workout. Each sheet will last you twenty-eight days—enough to carry you through a month of workouts.

Refer to the pages after these tables for descriptions, along with some finer points about the workouts and answers to the questions you may have.

For demos of all the exercises described here visit www.thenewprime/primetraining.

Beginner Strength Workouts

WORKOUT A

Movement Type	Exercise	Sets	Reps or Duration	Rest (Seconds)
Lower-body push	Front-Foot Elevated Static Lunge	2	15 (per leg)	60
Upper-body pull	Self-Assisted Pull-Up	2	15	60
Lower-body pull	Single-Leg Dead Lift	2	15 (per leg)	60
Upper-body push	Hands-Elevated Push-Up	2	15	60
Core	Push-Up Hold with Leg Lift	2	30–60 seconds	60

WORKOUT B

Movement Type	Exercise	Sets	Reps or Duration	Rest (Seconds)
Lower-body pull	Step-Up to Balance	2	15 (per leg)	60
Upper-body push	Single-Leg, Single-Arm Dumbbell Overhead Press	2	15 (per arm)	60
Lower-body push	Body-Weight Squat	2	As many as possible in 45 seconds	60
Upper-body pull	TRX Row	2	15	60
Core	Supine March	2	15 (per leg)	60

Exerciser Strength Workouts

WORKOUT A

Movement Type	Exercise	Sets	Reps or Duration	Rest (Seconds)
Lower-body push	Dynamic Lunge	3	10 per leg	45
Upper-body pull	Pull-Up or Assisted Pull-Up	3	10	45
Lower-body pull	Dead Lift	3	8	45
Upper-body push	Dumbbell Incline Bench Press	3	10	45
Core	Stir the Pot	3	10 per direction	45

WORKOUT B

Movement Type	Exercise	Sets	Reps or Duration	Rest (Seconds)
Lower-body pull	Step-Up to Reverse Lunge	3	10 per leg	45
Upper-body push	Dumbbell Overhead Press	3	10	45
Lower-body push	Barbell Squat	3	8	45
Upper-body pull	TRX Row, Feet Elevated, or TRX Row	3	10	45
Core	One-Arm Push-Up Hold	3	30 seconds per side	30

Athlete Strength Workouts

WORKOUT A

Movement Type	Exercise	Sets	Reps or Duration	Rest (Seconds)
1A. Lower-body push	Rear-Foot Elevated Static Lunge	3	As many as possible in 30 seconds (per leg)	0
1B. Upper-body pull	Pull-Up	3	As many as possible	30
2A. Lower-body pull	Alternating Power Step-Up	3	As many as possible in 30 seconds	0
2B. Upper-body push	Feet-Elevated Push-Up	3	As many as possible in 30 seconds	30
Core	Mountain Climber	4	As many as possible in 20 seconds	15

WORKOUT B

Movement Type	Exercise	Sets	Reps or Duration	Rest (Seconds)
1A. Lower-body pull	Dead Lift	4	6	0
1B. Upper-body push	Barbell Bench Press	4	6	60
2A. Lower-body push	Static Lunge	4	6 (per leg)	0
2B. Upper-body pull	Weighted TRX Row, Feet Elevated	4	6	60
Core	Stability Ball Pike	3	12	30

YOUR WORKOUT LOG

Level:

Workout (circle one): A   B

Starting Date:

Ending Date:

Exercise	Date	Sets	Reps	Rest	SET 1 wt/reps	SET 2 wt/reps	SET 3 wt/reps	SET 4 wt/reps

HOW TO USE THE WORKOUT LOG

1. Copy the blank log page twice.

2. On one copy, fill in the exercises, sets, reps, and rest periods for workout A in your program. On the other copy, do the same for workout B.

3. Each time you go into the gym, mark the date of your workout.

4. During your workout, record the amount of weight and the number of reps you perform on each set in the columns marked "Set, wt./reps." For example, if you did ten reps with ninety-five pounds for your first set on the bench press, you'd write "95/10" in the column labeled "Set 1, wt./reps."

5. Strive to complete a few more reps or to use a little more weight on each exercise each week. When you can complete all of your target reps in each set of an exercise, increase the weight by five to ten pounds the following week.

6. The sample table below indicates how a guy doing the beginner program, workout B, might progress week-to-week in the first exercise:

Exercise	Date	Sets	Reps	Rest	SET 1 wt/reps	SET 2 wt/reps	SET 3 wt/reps	SET 4 wt/reps
	11/5	2	15	60	30/15	30/11		
	11/9	2	15	60	30/15	30/15		
Step Up to Balance	11/14	2	15	60	40/13	40/10		
	11/19	2	15	60	40/15	40/10		
		"	"	"				
		"	"	"				

(Note that because the beginner program only has him doing two sets of this move, he doesn't use all four SET columns in this table.)

EXERCISE DESCRIPTIONS

Lower-Body Pushing Exercises

Static Lunge

- Stand with your feet together and your torso upright, and take a long step forward with your right foot.
- Keeping your torso upright and your gaze forward, slowly bend both legs until your left knee comes close to the floor.
- Pause and reverse the movement, returning to the right-foot-forward position, and repeat.
- Complete all reps with your right foot forward before switching to your left.
- Use dumbbells for additional resistance if necessary.

Front-Foot Elevated Static Lunge

Perform the movement as described under "Static Lunge," only this time with your front foot on a step or box eight to twelve inches high placed in front of you.

Rear-Foot Elevated Static Lunge

Perform the movement as described under "Static Lunge," only this time with the ball of your rear foot on a step or box eight to twelve inches high placed behind you.

Body-Weight Squat

- With your feet parallel and placed slightly wider than shoulder-width apart, slowly bend your knees and hips, sitting back until the tops of your thighs are parallel to the floor, keeping your lower back in a natural arch throughout the movement.
- Reverse the move, slowly standing back up, and repeat.

Barbell Squat

- Place a loaded barbell in a squat rack at shoulder-height and stand facing it.
- Take an overhead grip on the bar, slightly wider than shoulder-width.
- Walk toward the bar and duck your head underneath it so that the bar rests on the muscles of your upper back (not on your spine!).
- Walk your feet directly underneath the bar, stand up, and walk back a few steps.
- With your feet parallel and slightly wider than shoulder-width, slowly bend your knees and hips, sitting back until the tops of your thighs are parallel to the floor, keeping your lower back in a natural arch throughout the movement.
- Reverse the move, slowly standing back up, and repeat.

Dynamic Lunge

- Stand with your feet together and your torso upright, and take a long step forward with your right foot.
- Keeping your torso upright and your gaze forward, slowly bend both legs until your left knee comes close to the floor.
- Pause and reverse the movement, pushing forcefully off your lead foot and returning to the starting, feet-together position.
- Complete all reps with your right foot forward before switching to your left.
- Use dumbbells for additional resistance if necessary.

Lower-Body Pulling Exercises

Step-Up to Balance

- Stand behind a knee-high box, bench, or step.
- Keeping your feet parallel and your torso upright, step onto the box with your right foot.
- Lift your left knee as high as possible and hold for a one-count.
- Step off the bench with your left foot, then your right foot.
- Repeat this four-step movement for the appropriate number of reps, rest, then perform the same number of reps stepping onto the box with your left foot first.

Alternating Power Step-Up

Push explosively through your lead (right) foot when you step onto the box, jumping into the air and landing with your left foot on the box and your right foot on the floor. Repeat for the appropriate number of reps, switching the position of your feet while in the air on each rep.

Dead Lift

- Load an Olympic barbell (that's the one with the thick ends) with a moderately heavy to heavy weight and stand with the bar against the front of your shins (you can also use heavy kettlebells).
- Bend at the knees and hip joints and take an overhand, shoulder-width grip on the bar.
- Lower your hips until they are beneath the level of your shoulders.
- Keeping your arms straight, your lower back in its natural arch, your chest up, and your head in alignment with your spine, slowly stand fully upright.
- Keeping your lower back in its natural arch, bend at the hips and knees, lowering the bar to the floor, and repeat.

Single-Leg Dead Lift

• Stand upright, holding a heavy dumbbell in your left hand.

• Shift your weight onto your right foot and lift your left foot slightly off the floor.

• Keeping your lower back in its natural arch, your hips and shoulders square to the floor, and the dumbbell in your left hand close to your right leg, slowly hinge forward on your right hip, bending your right knee slightly and lifting your left leg directly behind you until the dumbbell is close to the floor.

• Pause, reverse the movement, and repeat.

Step-Up to Reverse Lunge

• Stand behind a knee-high box, bench, or step.

• Keeping your feet parallel and your torso upright, step your right leg backward into a lunge position.

• Rise out of the lunge position, driving your right foot forward, and step onto the bench with your right leg.

• Push up, raising your left leg into a high-knee position.

• Reverse the movement, lowering your left leg all the way to the floor.

• Repeat this movement for the appropriate number of reps, rest, then perform the same number of reps stepping back into the lunge position with your left foot.

Upper-Body Pushing Exercises

Hands-Elevated Push-Up

• Place your hands on a stable elevated surface (a bench, a box, or a table works well—the higher the surface, the easier the exercise) and assume a push-up position—hands and feet slightly wider than shoulder-width apart, balls of your feet on the floor, arms locked out, and body straight from your heels to the top of your head.

• Keeping your body straight and your head in a neutral position, simultaneously bend your arms and retract your shoulder blades until your chest lightly touches the bench or box, or as far as possible without losing good form.

• Reverse the movement, pushing yourself back up to the starting position.

Feet-Elevated Push-Up

Perform the movement described under "Hands-Elevated Push-Up," this time with your feet on an elevated box, bench, or chair.

Dumbbell Overhead Press

- Stand upright holding two dumbbells at shoulder height, palms facing forward or slightly inward.
- Keeping your torso vertical, exhale and press the dumbbells to arm's length overhead.
- Slowly lower the dumbbells back to the starting position and repeat.

Single-Leg, Single-Arm Dumbbell Overhead Press

Perform the movement with a dumbbell in one hand while balancing on the opposite foot. Complete all reps on one side before switching to your opposite hand and foot.

Dumbbell Incline Bench Press

- Set an exercise bench at a shallow incline (thirty degrees or less).
- Lie back on the bench, feet flat on the floor, holding two medium-heavy dumbbells near your shoulders (you should feel a stretch across your upper chest in this position).
- Exhale forcefully as you press the dumbbells to arm's length above you.
- Reverse the movement under control and repeat for repetitions.

Barbell Bench Press

- Place a barbell in the uprights of a bench press station, load it with a medium-heavy weight, and lie back on the bench.
- Keeping your feet flat on the floor, grip the bar evenly about six inches wider than shoulder-width on each side, and press it off the uprights.
- Slowly lower the bar until it contacts your chest about halfway down your rib cage.
- Press the bar back to the starting position, pause, and repeat.
- Always use a spotter when bench-pressing heavy weights.

Upper-Body Pulling Exercises

TRX Row

(NOTE: The TRX is a pair of nylon straps with handles attached that hangs from the wall or ceiling. It is available at most gyms.)

- Standing a few feet behind the anchor point for a TRX (or equivalent), raise the handles to chest height and walk backward (while facing the anchor point) until the straps are taut.
- Keeping your arms extended, walk your feet forward slowly until your body forms about a forty-five-degree angle to the floor.

- Keeping your body straight, head to heels, and your head in a neutral position relative to your spine, simultaneously bend your arms and pull your shoulder blades back, lifting your chest as high as you can toward the anchor point.
- Pause, slowly reverse the movement, and repeat for reps.
- To make the move more difficult, start with your feet closer toward the anchor point; to make it easier, start with them farther away.

TRX Row, Feet Elevated

Perform the same movement as described earlier with your feet elevated on a box or bench. The higher your feet, the tougher the exercise.

Weighted TRX Row, Feet Elevated

Perform the same movement, feet elevated, with a barbell plate placed flat against your chest. Pause for a two-count at the top of each repetition.

Self-Assisted Pull-Ups

- Place a chair, box, or bench beneath a chin-up station, high enough so that when you stand on the bench and grasp the bar, your arms are bent.
- Stand on the box and assume an underhand grip—palms facing you—on the bar (if you can't reach the bar comfortably at this point, get a taller bench).
- Simultaneously jump upward and pull yourself up with your arms until your chin clears the top of the bar.
- Hold the top position for a one-count, then slowly lower yourself back down to the bench, bending your legs slightly until your arms extend fully.

Pull-Ups

Perform the movement as described under "Self-Assisted Pull-Ups," but without help from your legs, hanging freely beneath the bar and pulling yourself up using your upper body only. If possible, extend your arms fully between repetitions.

Core Exercises

Push-Up Hold with Leg Lift

- Assume a push-up position—hands and feet slightly wider than shoulder-width apart, balls of your feet on the floor, arms locked, and body straight from the heels to the top of your head.
- Keeping your body straight, and the toes of your right foot pointing toward the floor, slowly lift your right leg six inches off the floor, strongly contracting the right glute.
- Hold for five seconds.
- Slowly lower the right leg to the floor and repeat, alternating feet on each rep.

Supine March

- Lie on your back with your legs bent, your feet flat on the floor, and your arms on the floor, palms-down.
- Draw your right knee toward your chest and simultaneously push your left foot into the floor, lifting your pelvis as high as you can.
- Strongly contract your left glute for a one-count, lower your pelvis, and repeat on the opposite side, alternating sides until you have completed the appropriate number of reps on each side.

Stir the Pot

- Assume a "plank" position with your forearms and hands resting on a stability ball, your upper body straight from your heels to the top of your head, and your lower back in its natural arch.
- Keeping your body rigid and your head in a neutral position relative to the floor, circle your elbows as widely and slowly as possible in a clockwise direction.
- After completing a full clockwise circle, perform the same movement counterclockwise.
- Continue alternating the direction of the circle on each rep until you have completed all the reps in your set.

One-Arm Push-Up Hold

- Assume a push-up position.
- Keeping your hips and shoulders level with the floor, raise one arm from the floor and put it behind your back.
- Hold for thirty seconds, switch arms, and repeat.

Mountain Climber

From the push-up position, draw your right knee quickly toward your chest, then return it to the starting position. Alternate sides as fast as possible for a set period or number of reps.

Stability Ball Pike

- Assume a push-up position—hands and feet slightly wider than shoulder-width apart, balls of your feet on the floor, arms locked, and body straight from your heels to the top of your head— with your feet elevated on a stability ball.
- Keeping your arms and legs straight, contract your core musculature, lifting your hips as high in the air as possible (the ball will roll toward you)
- Hold for a moment, squeezing your abdomen as much as possible, then reverse the movement and slowly return to the starting position.

Answers to Questions I Know You'll Have about the Strength Programs

1. What is with the "1A" and "1B" notation on the athlete-level workouts?

1A and 1B, and 2A and 2B indicate that the two exercises that share a number are "paired," meaning that you perform a set of the first exercise (1A or 2A) and then, with minimal rest, a set of the second exercise (1B or 2B). You then rest for the time indicated and then return to the first exercise.

Pairing exercises naturally makes a workout more intense because you rest less and move more during your time in the gym. Simultaneously, though, each muscle group gets more rest between efforts. This turns your strength workout into a bit of a cardio challenge as well, embracing more of my "work the whole body at once" philosophy.

2. How do I handle rest periods on single-leg or single-arm movements?

On a movement like the static lunge (athlete level, workout B), you perform all your reps for the first leg (six in this case), rest minimally while you change legs, and perform all your reps on the other leg. On the single-leg, single-arm dumbbell overhead press (beginner level, workout B) it's the same approach: do all your reps on one side, then rest minimally while you switch the dumbbell to your other hand, and do the reps on that side.

3. Some of the tables say "As many as possible" or "As many as possible in 30 seconds." Please explain.

On those exercises, rather than perform a set number of repetitions, you'll do either *as many as you can without breaking form* or *as many as you can in the time indicated*. So if you're doing pull-ups (as in the exerciser program, workout A), you'll hang from the bar and simply do as many reps as you can without stopping—just like in gym class way back when. If you're doing alternating power step-ups (as in the athlete program, workout A), you'll stand near a clock (or use a stopwatch or other timer) and blast out as many reps of the move as you can, using good form, in thirty seconds.

In the first type of exercise, you'll work at a deliberate pace—not too fast, not too slow. In the second, you work as fast and explosively as you can while maintaining good form.

How much weight should I use?

Ah, the eternal question. If you've never lifted weights before, or are unfamiliar with the movements described, always be conservative at first. Start with a weight you know you can handle and work up to something more challenging as your thirty-day period goes on.

That said, remember that to be effective, strength training needs to be *progressive*: if you're not doing a little bit more—or at least trying to—in the gym, one day to the next, you're not working hard enough. Strive to add a rep or two, or a pound or five, to each exercise, each time you do it. You can "hack" this process a little by starting out each new phase using weights that are slightly less than you think you can handle, and finishing each phase using weights that are slightly *more* than you initially thought you could handle.

Here's how that might work in practice. Let's say you're doing the exerciser program. And let's say that from past experience, you know that within the last six months or so you dead-lifted 155 pounds for twelve reps with a fair amount of effort.

You might start your thirty-day program working with 135—knowing that you'll be trying to increase the weight steadily over a four-week period. If you dead lift once or twice a week and increase the weight by just five pounds per workout, that would bring your dead lift up to 165 pounds for three sets of eight to twelve reps by the end of the phase—a pretty solid accomplishment.

Now, regular lifters know that steady, long-term incremental strength improvement—even in this peak-and-back-off wave pattern—are mostly the domain of newbies, steroid users, and genetic freaks. A five-pound increase per week over several weeks, even on a big-ticket move like a dead lift, is a high bar to shoot for. But your intention should always be to hit new heights at the end of each cycle—even if it's just one extra rep at the same weight with good form. For a guy with experience, that's progress enough.

How do I know when to add weight?

When you can perform all your target reps on all the prescribed sets for a given exercise, that's when you increase weight—by as small an increment as possible.

For barbell exercises, that should be five pounds. You may have to scour the gym for the two-and-a-half-pound plates, but you'll find them.

Most gyms have dumbbells that go up in five-pound increments. For upper-body moves, that means you'll need to make a ten-pound jump each time you hit your target sets and reps—a big jump but doable. For lower-body moves, however, such as the dynamic lunge or step-up, you can hold a slightly heavier dumbbell in one hand than the other—a twenty-five in your right hand and a twenty in your left, for example—which allows you to increase the weight you use a little more slowly. That's always a good thing. Place the heavier weight in a different hand each set. Be ready for helpful gym rats to tell you, repeatedly, that your dumbbells don't match.

Some of these movements feel uncomfortable and hurt my joints. Can I do something else instead?

Some gym-goers will insist that certain exercises have near-magical powers to confer gains in strength and muscle. The barbell squat, in particular, seems to get lots of acclaim as "the king of exercises," followed closely by the dead lift (with lesser subjects like the barbell bent row serving as trusted advisers, and lowly isolation moves like triceps kickbacks working menial jobs as chambermaids and court jesters). I'll leave it to the Internet warriors to hash out the relative merits of all these moves, but for an over-forty guy like you, the number one factor in choosing exercises should be *ease and comfort of execution.*

That probably sounds like an oxymoron, since we're talking about lifting heavy objects over and over again, an inherently uncomfortable endeavor. What I mean is that every movement you do in the weight room should feel athletic, smooth, controlled, and coordinated. You shouldn't feel—or look, if you're using the gym mirror—like Quasimodo shambling up the clock tower stairs. If your knees, lower back, elbows, neck, or some other area is complaining while you do a move, even though you've completed a thorough warm-up beforehand, find another move. (Find one in the same movement category, naturally: don't substitute a core move for an upper-body push move.) You can use the ones in this book, search my site (www.thenewprime.com/primetraining), or ask a trainer at your gym for an alternative.

As each set progresses, you will probably feel a burning sensation in your muscles. But if you feel it in your joints, there's something wrong. Back off and try another move.

I don't see any curls or triceps extensions in this program. Will I wind up with skinny arms?
It's true: I include exactly zero direct arm work in this program: no barbell curls, no triceps push-downs.

It isn't that those moves are *totally* useless. It's that they're redundant.

When you do a row or a chin-up exercise, your biceps muscles work hard to help you pull your chest or chin toward the bar, or vice versa. And when you do a push-up or an overhead press, your triceps labor mightily to help push yourself—or the bar—skyward. These muscles actually work *harder* helping your bigger muscles move the larger loads than they do when you do curls, extensions, or other such vanity-enhancing fare.

Your arm muscles get plenty of work in this program, believe me. If you have the genetics to build huge guns, this program will get you there.

However, I will make one concession to guys who really care about how their arms look in a T-shirt (and I sympathize): go ahead and do some curls and extensions at the end of the workout. Give yourself *five minutes*—no more—to do whatever babe-magnet move you want before you towel off and leave the gym. It won't help your functional fitness much, but it certainly won't kill you. And if the eighth-of-an-inch of extra vein definition you get out of it will be met approvingly by your wife or partner, well, mission accomplished.

What am I supposed to do after thirty days?

After the thirty-day period is up, you have a number of options. One is to switch to the next phase: beginners to exercisers, and exercisers to athletes. What you've done this month has prepared you for what comes next.

Athletes can benefit from cycling back to the beginner program for a thirty-day period, then following that up with thirty days on the exerciser program. Your body will thank you for the lower resistance and slightly less challenging moves. If you like, you can always increase the weight or add a set or two to make the lower-level programs more challenging, but don't knock them till you try them: in Your New Prime workout program, even the beginner program is challenging—and you may need it after pounding through the athlete program for a month.

Another option after your first thirty days is to explore my website, www.thenewprime. com/primetraining, for other ideas and workouts you can do as you get fitter and more comfortable with the exercises.

Finally, you can also strike out on your own: hire a trainer or go in with a buddy on one and work out together, or explore other online resources or books. These thirty days are only the beginning.

HOW NOT TO GET FIT: CYCLING

Not long ago I took a leisurely bike ride with a group that included a fanatical cyclist. He knew everything about bikes: wind resistance, optimal posture, component weight. A dyed-in-the-wool bike nerd.

At one point during our ride, he announced to the group that he frequently did sixty-mile training rides. This was up from twenty-five or thirty miles at a time a year or two before. His rides would take hours. That very day, in fact, when the rest of us in the cycling group were planning on calling it quits, he planned on cycling another fifteen miles home.

I have to give the man points for dedication, but despite all his efforts, he was frustrated because he had a sizeable gut; he admitted that no matter how far he rode, he couldn't seem to lose it.

Moments before, he had told us he had dropped a thousand bucks on a new gear system to save himself just under a half pound of bike weight. He said it made his hill climbs easier.

I felt bad for the guy, but I wasn't altogether surprised about his weight problem, either. Genetics plays a role in the ease or difficulty of burning off flab. But choosing long, slow cycling as your primary form of exercise activity doesn't help.

When you ride a bike, after all, your weight is supported entirely by a metal frame. Your body absorbs no impact. Your legs work hard, granted, but in a very limited, extremely repetitive range of motion in a movement that isn't particularly organic. And because your legs never actually support your weight or absorb any force from the ground, your bones aren't stimulated to grow and thicken, and your muscles don't undergo *eccentric* contraction—that is, they never lengthen under tension, which is a key factor in muscle growth.

And fast, hard muscle contraction, not long, slow cardio, is what drives fat loss. The more muscle you have, the bigger and hotter your fat-burning engine. The less you have, the more likely you'll wind up "skinny-fat": paunchy with no noticeable muscle development, like the unfortunate cyclist I went out with that day.

Still another problem: cycling puts you in the dreaded sitting position—something we all do far too much of anyway. It also seems to inspire in its participants an overwhelming urge to make repeated pit stops at Starbucks for thousand-calorie Frappuccinos and muffins, figuring their easy cruise through town will burn it all off.

This is all on top of erectile issues and prostate problems, which can result from too much cycling on the wrong kind of seat (more on this in chapter 5).

Look, if you adore cycling, do it—in moderation. Personally, I love mountain biking, which is typically more intense than road biking, and I fully approve of cycle commuting, as long as you're able to stay safe and avoid busy streets (where I live, new "ghost bikes"—white painted bike frames chained to a post near the site of a fatal bike crash—pop up every few months). A long ride on the weekend or an outing with your son or daughter as part of an "active rest" day can be a lot of fun: you'll be out in the fresh air, after all, easily moving along at a speed far faster than you can comfortably run. And high-intensity work on a bike—fast, hard hill climbs and sprints in a high gear—can be great for you.

But unless you're seriously out of shape, don't expect long, leisurely rides to build any muscle or put much of a dent in your fat stores. Don't ride in lieu of strength training, mobility work, foam rolling, or a PRIME Workout. And don't ride for exceptional fitness. Ride for enjoyment, relaxation, and social connection—all of which are invaluable.

BUILDING ENDURANCE WITH PRIME WORKOUTS

Sunday	Monday	Tuesday	Wednesday	Thursday	Friday	Saturday
Active rest	Mobility program	Mobility program	Mobility program	Fun activity, ideally outdoors	Mobility program	Mobility program
	Strength workout A	**PRIME Workout**	Strength workout B		Strength workout A	**PRIME Workout**

The final component of Your New Prime workout program is your PRIME Workouts: peak repetition intervals with maximum effort, which are my personalized take on high-intensity interval training (HIIT).

This style of training has received tons of attention in the news in the last few years, and with good reason. Back in the nineties, the prevailing wisdom was that if you wanted to develop cardiovascular fitness, you had to do tons of slow, steady-state repetitive exercise like jogging or cycling. By the 2000s, research caught up to what some trainers had discovered intuitively nearly one hundred years before: that much the same results (and in many ways better results) could be had with a much smaller investment of time. One 2012 study found that just six interval workouts, totaling just a few minutes each, produced measurable improvements in key markers of cardiovascular health.

I've already laid out my argument that that long, slow cardio is not the best use of your training time: the repetitive movement is hell on your joints. It's inefficient, timewise; and—subjectively, I concede—it's not as fun as sprint work. Compared with PRIME Workouts, long, slow cardio is also not an efficient fat-burner. Consistently, people who do tons of jogging and cycling do not lose a lot of fat—especially in comparison with the amount of time they spend running and cycling. But people who sprint burn a *ton* of fat, relatively speaking. For cardio health, body composition, and joint health, PRIME training is a win-win-win. And with the flexibility and adaptability of these workouts, you'll never get bored. You never even have to repeat the same cardiovascular workout twice if you don't want to. Ever.

Here's how to put together a PRIME Workout:

Choose Activities and Set Them Up

Choose two to three different activities and set them up in a circuit (a set sequence). Weight-bearing moves like sprinting, hill running, rope jumping, beach sprints, and stadium runs are probably the toughest and most effective, but PRIME Workouts are effective with virtually any challenging physical activity you can safely keep up for about thirty seconds. You could also choose burpees, jumping jacks, body weight exercises, or mountain biking. Traditional cardio machines like the elliptical trainer, Stepmill, or stationary bike work great, too, with the added advantage of being low-impact and therefore very safe for beginners.

If you choose body weight strength moves, *don't* choose movements that isolate a single muscle group like curls, lateral raises, or triceps extensions—they won't work enough muscle tissue to challenge your cardiovascular system. Choose instead moves like bodyweight squats, push-ups, burpees, jumps, and, if you're really tough, pull-ups.

Whatever moves you choose, let them be exercises you enjoy, can do with good form, and can perform relatively easily at the gym or wherever you're exercising (don't choose to use both the rower and the treadmill in your workout if those two pieces of equipment are fifty yards away from one another at your gym!). Most important, choose movements you can do without hurting yourself. If you have a bad knee or a bum lower back, whatever you do, don't pick moves that will bother them. You need an activity that's safe for you at a high intensity. The Stepmill and stationary bike work well for most people, and the weighted sled push, at thirty-second intervals, and the diabolical Versaclimber, at twenty-second intervals, are my all-time personal favorites.

Why is it so important that the exercises be moves you can do with good form?

Because you're going to do them *as hard as you can*. PRIME Workouts are *tough*. I can't stress this enough. It's not easy cardio, light strength training, or jogging. It's as fast and furious as you can go.

Choose a Work-Rest Time Interval

Once you've picked your exercises for the day, choose a work-rest time interval. For example, thirty seconds on, ninety seconds off works very well for tougher exercises, but forty-five seconds, seventy-five seconds is reasonable, and one minute, two minutes—though painful—can work well too. Some athletic types who enjoy explosive sports can even go for *very* short intervals of ten to twelve seconds, with rest of up to forty seconds between efforts, so they can ensure a fast and furious pace during those work intervals. With PRIME Workouts, it's up to you.

Beginners, naturally enough, do well working less and resting slightly more in their PRIME Workouts, and so they should choose a work-to-rest interval of 1:2 or even 1:3 (for example, thirty seconds of work followed by sixty or ninety seconds of rest). As you get better, you may choose to work more, and rest less—say, forty-five seconds of work followed by a brief fifteen seconds of rest. This would be an interval to shoot for by the time you reach the athlete level.

With most activities, longer intervals (over one minute) are less effective than shorter ones, as you want to be able to work at or close to your maximum intensity for the whole work interval. Physiologically, you can't redline it for more than a minute at a time; your body will run out of the high-performance fuel necessary for max-effort sprinting before the one-minute mark.

Choose the Number of Reps

At first, choosing the number of reps for the circuit will be determined by your fitness level: PRIME Workouts are tough, and your first few times out, you may get only one or two circuits in before you become exhausted, or even start to feel a little woozy. Soon enough, though, you'll be able to crank out up to a half dozen circuits at full throttle. In my experience, four to eight rounds of the hardest, weight-bearing activities are plenty for even very fit guys. If you're doing shorter intervals (ten to twelve seconds), or working on a bike or a piece of weight-bearing cardio equipment, you can do up to twelve. That's fine, as long as you stick to my PRIME Workout rules, which are pretty simple:

- Warm up thoroughly, using the foam rolling and mobility moves described in the mobility program.

- Perform each interval at maximum intensity.

- Stop your workout if you feel dizzy or nauseated, or if you have joint pain.

- If you're wearing a heart rate monitor, your heart rate should reach 90 to 100 percent of your maximum heart rate during (or directly after) your work intervals.

- Stop your workout if your speed in any individual interval drops by more than 10 percent.

With so many different activities and different work/rest intervals to choose from, each of which places a slightly different demand on your muscles, joints, cardiovascular system, and nervous system, there's never a reason to get bored—or hurt—doing these workouts. Variety will be your saving grace in staying healthy, fit, and strong.

PRIME Workout Samples

Here are a few PRIME Workout samples for each experience level. Adjust the duration and rest times according to your fitness level—and don't forget to warm up!

BEGINNER-LEVEL PRIME WORKOUT: GYM OPTION

Exercise	Work Interval (Seconds)	Rest Interval (Seconds)
Stationary Bike	30	60
Rowing Machine	30	60
Dynamic Lunge	30	60

Repeat entire sequence a total of three times.

BEGINNER-LEVEL PRIME WORKOUT: OUTDOOR OPTION

Exercise	Work Interval (Seconds)	Rest Interval (Seconds)
Bodyweight Squat	30	90
Jumping Jack	30	90
Run/Sprint	30	90

Repeat entire sequence a total of three to six times.

EXERCISER-LEVEL PRIME WORKOUT: GYM OPTION

Exercise	Work Interval (Seconds)	Rest Interval (Seconds)
Versaclimber	20	60
Box Jump	20	60
Push-Ups	20 (or until failure)	60

Repeat entire sequence a total of four to eight times.

EXERCISER-LEVEL PRIME WORKOUT: OUTDOOR TRACK/TRAIL RUNNING OPTION

1. Warm-up: easy run, one quarter mile
2. Thirty-second run, 30 percent effort (light jog)
3. Fifteen-second run, 70 percent effort (a level at which talking is difficult)
4. Ten-second sprint, 90–100 percent effort (maximum effort)
5. Two minutes' rest

Repeat steps two through five continuously, for a total of at least four times.

ATHLETE-LEVEL PRIME WORKOUT: GYM OPTION

Exercise	Work Interval (Seconds)	Rest Interval (Seconds)
Body-Weight Squat	30	15
Jump Rope	150 Revolutions	15
Push-Up	30	15

Repeat entire sequence a total of three to five times.

ATHLETE-LEVEL PRIME WORKOUT: OUTDOOR OPTION

Exercise	Work Interval (Seconds)	Rest Interval (Seconds)
Bear Crawl	45	15
Hill Run	45	15
Jump Rope	45	15

Repeat entire sequence a total of three to five times.

ATHLETE-LEVEL PRIME WORKOUT: BEACH OPTION

Exercise	Work Interval (Seconds)	Rest Interval (Seconds)
Beach Sprint	30	60
In-and-Out*	As Fast as Possible	60
Burpees	30	60

*Run into the water, swim past the breakers, and bodysurf back to shore, as fast as you can.

Repeat entire sequence a total of three to five times.

Personally, I love putting together "freestyle" PRIME Workouts based on whatever is available in my workout environment, as with the beach workout described earlier. If I'm out for a run in a place I don't know well, and I happen upon a park bench or a steep hill or a set of stairs, I might stop and do thirty seconds of bench step-ups or a stair sprint or a hill run—all to keep my mind engaged, and my body guessing and adapting. Another option, if you have access to a park, is to set up a thirty-second obstacle course that requires a *combination* of climbing, crawling, jumping, and sprinting, and slam through the whole thing eight to ten times, resting a minute or so between efforts. Exhausting and exhilarating.

For a few more of my favorite PRIME exercises and workouts, check out www.thenew prime.com/primetraining.

HOW NOT TO GET FIT: GOLF, WALKING YOUR DOG, PLAYING CATCH

I come across this situation far more often than I'd like. Someone will call me up looking for wellness advice. They'll ask me about supplements, stress control, nutrition, sleep. They'll go into great detail, wondering what they can do to fix whatever ails them, and I'll do my best to respond.

At some point I'll ask them what they do for exercise.

"Of course I exercise!" they say. "I walk my dog twice a day!"

Or, just as bad, "I play golf on the weekends!"

I want to jump through the phone and strangle them.

Once more, with feeling: low-intensity movements that involve mostly walking aren't "exercise." They're NEAT: non–exercise activity thermogenesis.

That doesn't mean they aren't good uses of your time. Taking your dog for a walk is great for you, Spot, and Spot's bladder. But stop thinking of a leisurely stroll as an exercise program.

Want to take Spot for a half dozen uphill sprints (which he'd probably love)? That's a different story. Or hike up a mountain carrying thirty pounds of gear? Now you're talking.

Golf isn't a workout. It's a pleasant way to pass a sunny afternoon. That's why golf pros can do it in pressed pants and polo shirts: they're in no danger of sweating through them. If tons of NEAT is all you can get in a given day (especially an off-day from exercise), it's far better than doing nothing at all. But don't expect it to reshape your body, build any muscle, or prevent you from otherwise sliding into middle-aged decrepitude in any meaningful way.

What to Do on Your "Off-Days"

Sunday	Monday	Tuesday	Wednesday	Thursday	Friday	Saturday
Active rest	Mobility program	Mobility program	Mobility program	**Fun activity, ideally outdoors**	Mobility program	Mobility program
	Strength workout A	PRIME Workout	Strength workout B		Strength workout A	PRIME Workout

I'll come clean: I don't believe in "off-days."

In any given week on Your New Prime workout program, you'll have two days that are less structured than the others. As I've noted, you'll want to spend them in the following way:

- Your *fun activity* day (Thursday for our sample guy), on which you should do some fairly intense but fun activity, such as a sport or a strenuous hike.

- Your *active rest* day (Sunday for our guy), which you should spend on less taxing movements. Think fun activities like surfing, paddleboarding, or mountain biking if you can get outside, some easy lap swimming or treadmill trotting if you can't.

Whereas you may be dripping with sweat after your "fun" day playing racquetball or basketball with friends, you may just get a light gloss on your active rest day. But both days should be *fun*—one just a little more "serious fun" than the other. It's quite possible that what you now consider "exercise" will be demoted to "non-exercise activity" on your off-days. Those are the days you celebrate and use your newfound fitness!

As you no doubt know by now, I'm a movement freak and I believe you should move as much as possible. A trainer I know takes his clients' vital signs before every workout and has found that those who sat on the couch all weekend typically have the worst readings on Mondays. So get moving, even—maybe especially—on those "off-days."

BOXING: THE EXERCISE I'D DO IF IT WAS ALL I COULD DO

If you were to ask me what type of exercise I consider the most complete, most challenging, and most fun, I'd give an answer that might surprise you.

Boxing.

Boxing develops the athletic trifecta of strength, power, and stamina. Since it requires you to move in all directions—up, down, forward, back, twisting left and right—it enhances mobility as well. It's a skill you can continue to refine throughout your life, and it even has real-world applications (should the need arise).

Primarily, though, I love the elemental quality of boxing. When you're sparring, you're putting all your physical and mental skills to work to score a victory against an opponent who's trying to do the same to you. When you're working with a trainer, he's doing everything he can to push and challenge you, and you're doing everything you can to keep up. John Snow, my boxing trainer at NYC's Trinity Boxing Club, talks about boxing as a metaphor for life: whether you're sparring or simply training, you have to man up, face your fears, and go to work.

In my many years of doing athletics of all kinds, I've never encountered an activity that is so thoroughly exhausting as hitting a heavy bag or hitting focus mitts with a demanding trainer. Something about putting every ounce of your power into punching combinations—over and over and over again—for three long minutes, all while shuffling around, dodging blows, and listening to the trainer's commands, takes everything out of me. And at the end of the workout, I feel clean, clear, reborn. On top of everything else, boxing is a great stress-buster.

I'll never stop doing strength and cardio work. The foundation of general fitness that those activities provide is what allows me to go into John's gym whenever I'm in New York City and mix it up without throwing my back out or giving myself a heart attack. But boxing makes my heart pound, and not just because it's great exercise. To me, it puts me in the headspace where I want to live my life: excited, intensely focused, fired-up, and ready for anything.

The Rocky movies didn't rake in over a billion dollars at the box office because they're about boxing. It's because they were about spiritual transformation through physical effort. That's what we're all after when we go to the gym. That's why we continue to go—even long after we've achieved the minimal baseline of health and fitness that keeps our doctors happy.

Boxing may do this for you, as it does for me—or it may not. But *some* physical sport or activity will. Once you developed a solid base of fitness on Your New Prime workout program—and that won't take long, believe me—I advise you to find it. And then do it whenever you can, like your life depends on it.

SIX REASONS TO LOVE THE 5K

The marathon (and the Ironman triathlon) have developed a reputation as the true test of athletic fortitude: manhood in 26.2 miles. Buy into this myth too completely, however, and you may end up hurting yourself.

My suggestion? Embrace the 5K.

Why do I love the five-kilometer (3.1-mile) distance so much? Let me count the ways.

1. Anyone Can Do It

A very unfit person can still walk 5K—or at least work up to walking 5K in a matter of a few weeks. It won't wreck that unfit person the way a marathon will. And it won't require an investment of time that's unavailable to 99 percent of the population (the way an Ironman or a marathon will). The entry point, in other words, is accessible.

2. It Offers a Challenge to Everyone

An unfit desk-jockey guy with three months of training to his name will be ecstatic to simply *finish* a 5K. But even the fittest guy you know can keep working on his 5K time, forever. It doesn't matter who you are—running three miles as fast as you can is *exhausting*. It's plenty of workout for one day. If I were a betting man, I'd stake my whole year's salary that the average guy running a sub-19:30 5K is healthier than the average guy running a sub-four-hour marathon. Get faster at the 5K, and it's a pretty good bet you've gotten healthier all around. Get faster at a marathon and you may well have gotten *unhealthier*.

3. You Can Still Have a Life

Even if you make 5K training the center of your exercise life (by running, say, a half-dozen races a year—not a bad way of organizing these things, if you ask me), you don't have to obsess. You don't have to put in three hours of junk miles before work. You can make great progress on your 5K time by running just two or three times a week for less than an hour. You're training for a race that will take under a half hour, after all.

4. You Can Race Whenever You Want To

Although marathons are getting more and more common (there were over 1,100 marathons in the United States in 2013), you still have to wait around—and possibly travel—to get to one. And unless you're pathological, you wouldn't want to do more than a handful in the span of a single year anyway. 5Ks, however, are far more ubiquitous. There are 5Ks to support charities, fun-run 5Ks that families can do together, 5Ks to raise awareness for . . . well . . . just about anything. They happen almost every weekend. And since they won't break your body down in the same way that a marathon will, you don't have to wait weeks between races if you don't want to. You could conservatively race three times in a single month and expect to approach your best times in each one.

5. The Training Is Better for You

As I pointed out, training for a long-distance race tends to do bad things for your health. But training for a 5K does the opposite: you'll be in that beneficial pocket of ten miles a week (maximum), two to three workouts a week. And once you've passed the early phases of training, at least some of those workouts will be speed workouts—meaning you'll be stimulating your type II (strength and power) muscle fibers. That's something long, slow distance training won't do for you. And since your workouts will take less than an hour (sometimes much less), you'll be doing good things for your hormonal profile at the same time by upping testosterone and HGH. Another benefit? You don't have to chug down sugary drinks, gels, and bars to make it through a 5K as you do for a marathon. You can eat healthier and still finish fast.

6. Competing Is Good

So you're sold on the benefits of the 5K distance, and you work on your speed. You feel fast, you feel in the groove. To my mind, you haven't closed the loop until you've actually slapped down the money to enter the race and posted an official time in an official race against others who have been doing the same thing.

Sound like a superficial difference? It isn't. From personal experience, I can tell you it's great to toe the line with a few dozen other racers, all of whom have been working for at least as long as you have to get to that point. Since you're usually separated by age and gender, you'll be penned up with fellow forty-plus guys (to whom you can recommend this book). The camaraderie is palpable, and you may start to run into the same guys at these events and even kick off a friendship or two.

And then, once you complete your race, there's nothing like seeing your name posted in black and white in the top twenty or so finishers. Then in the top ten. Then the top five. Then maybe on the medal podium.

It can be done. Much more easily—and less painfully—than finishing that high in your local marathon.

YOUR THIRTY-DAY ACTION PLAN FOR FUNCTIONAL FITNESS

1. **Get rolling on the fitness program.** Figure out what level you're at, then get moving on the mobility/strength/endurance program as outlined. Choose a start date and get to it.

2. **NEAT-en up.** Start looking for ways to get more movement into your day: Pace while you talk on the phone. Do push-ups during commercial breaks.

3. **Stop being your own worst enemy.** As many reasons as there are to work out—and your average trainer can rattle off a few dozen—somehow we guys can come up with ten more not to. Get in the habit. Unless you're at death's door, make it non-negotiable.

4. **Get out of your chair.** Every fifteen minutes, get up from your desk chair. Better yet, start spending at least part of your day standing (or walking) while you work.

5. **Ease up on the long-distance work.** If you're a runner or a cyclist, consider easing back on those activities. Don't skip them altogether if you enjoy them— just begin prioritizing higher-intensity activities.

6. **Sign up for a 5K (or a mud run, or an obstacle course race, or an ocean swim).** Most guys should be able to at least complete a 5K with a combination of running and walking after at most three months of training. Look ahead in the calendar, find an event (active.com is a great source!), and sign up to mark your first ninety days on your fitness program.

7. **Eyes off the mirror, feet off the scale.** Fitness is about functioning well. If you focus on that—improving your performance in the areas of strength, mobility, and endurance—you'll look better and your weight will come closer to optimal on its own. Obsessing over how you look and how much you weigh is taking your eye off the ball.

8. **Steal workouts.** Look for ways during social events, weekend getaways, and other gatherings to throw in some type of movement. Walk the beach, a trail, or a wooded path while catching up with friends. Toss a ball with your son or daughter. Bike to lunch with your wife. These aren't workouts—they're just activities that fit people (like you) do for fun.

PART III

SEX, STRESS, AND OTHER CONFUSING STUFF

Tuning Up Your Brain— and Your Balls— for the Long Game

CHAPTER 5

Life Below the Belt

Sex in Your New Prime

GREAT EXPECTATIONS

If we talk about it at all, we guys tend to discuss sex like we're talking about sports. Stats and measures, averages and at bats, whether we scored, whether we *could* score, and if not, what base we reached or might reach, and with what type of partner. Many of us view it as another game, another way to compete with one another, and, perhaps more important, another way to measure ourselves in that everlasting self-check that runs through our minds all day, every day. While unfair, sexual partners are often thought of as a reflection of us— like a car or a bank balance—and their level of desire for us is an affirmation of, or an affront to, who we are.

It's not exactly the most enlightened view of sex, but it's easy to see where those feelings may come from. The media is chock-full of images of handsome, rich, superfit guys with supermodels or actresses on their arms. When sex happens to these superheroes—think Brad Pitt and Angelina Jolie in *Mr. and Mrs. Smith*—it's *rapturous*: someone is sprawled on a kitchen table, both parties are so excited they chew through one another's clothes, and they run through every sex act imaginable (while improvising a few new ones along the way). The stars align, the angels sing, a screaming guitar solo shakes the rafters, and the whole thing ends with such explosive force that the neighbors think an atom bomb has detonated next door.

That's how it's supposed to go down every night. Twice a night. Forever!

And of course all this rapture is supposed to happen without talking about it. Ever. We don't tell our partners that we might be bored with how things are going in the bedroom; we don't go near the topic of unexpressed desires or fantasies. Maybe we're a little ashamed of them, even, and figure they're better left unsaid. We assume our partners, for their part, must be fine—their needs are being met with the occasional "safe" sex that you're having. Surely they'd say something if it were otherwise . . . right?

With poor communication and sky-high expectations serving as a backdrop, is it any wonder that so many older men—57 percent, according to a recent survey—report that they are unhappy with their sex lives? Up to one in five cases of erectile dysfunction are purely psychological—caused by stress, performance anxiety, and the myriad other demons that float through our gray matter on a regular basis. Might the ongoing head trip of BS that we consume from the media about how sex is supposed to happen between consenting adults be at least partially responsible for the pervasiveness of erectile dysfunction? ED levels are currently around 30 percent among fifty-year-olds.

Add to this the fact that our old friends obesity, stress (particularly financial stress), diabetes, depression, and heart disease—rampant in today's culture—all substantially increase the risk of ED, and you have a veritable perfect storm for pervasive male sexual dissatisfaction and dysfunction. It's a wonder anyone is getting it up, much less getting it on, in this day and age.

To remind you: I'm not a doctor or a therapist. But I'm familiar with the problems my fellow men over forty face in the bedroom, and the virility-sapping environment in which we're all immersed. I hear about the sexual problems men my age have all the time: waning desire and performance; lack of excitement, adventurousness, and spontaneity; lack of real connection; physical limitations; self-image issues; extramarital wanderings; porn addiction—and the list goes on.

As a guy with twenty-seven years and counting in the trenches of a strong, passionate marriage, I'm here to tell you that what we see every day in the media about how a marriage is supposed to work—endless desire, perfect harmony, everlasting respect and support, all without a shred of effort or attention on anyone's part—is a myth. That James Bond–esque guy we all think we're supposed to be doesn't exist. In the real world, a chain-smoking boozer like Bond would probably have gonorrhea, a potbelly, and issues with impotence.

That doesn't mean, however, that guys over forty can't get much, much more out of their sex lives than they currently do. But to do that we've got to face up to the issue that plagues our long-term relationships the most: complacency.

In the same way that complacency threatens our careers, health, finances, fitness, and relationships with others, it also threatens our sex lives. Unless we constantly reinvest passion and commitment into our health, professions, diets, physiques, and, yes, sexual relationships, we get resigned. We figure that things have peaked, that it can't get any better and is likely to get only worse. Instead of trying to improve things, we decide we're going to ride it out, just the way it is, all the way till the bitter end.

Don't even think about it, New Primer.

As with all these other aspects of your life, you can get more—not less—out of your sex life as you get older *if* you take immaculate care of your health, inside and out, and reconnect with the passion, mystery, creativity, and urgency that started your relationship in the first place (however well-worn or nascent it may be). Maybe you won't have the stamina and drive you had when you were a teenager, but you will have something that I believe is better: a passionate relationship that feels both secure and adventurous at the same time.

That's a big promise. So how do you do it?

I'm going to spell things out for you in plain terms in this chapter. As you'll see, the material is broken up into subheadings based on the common issues that most men face in their sex lives as they approach, and pass, the forty-year mark. One at a time, I'm going to go through each of these issues and show you how you can conquer them.

The chapter is broken cleanly into two main parts: *psychological* issues and *physical* issues. That's because, as you know, sex is neither purely a matter of mechanics nor purely a matter of emotions. It's in that mysterious meeting place between body and mind. Both need to be fully on board to get the job done. This chapter will show you techniques you can start to implement in the next thirty days to make that happen.

Fair warning: this chapter gets a little blue. There's no way around straight talk when you're discussing sexual matters. I urge you to plow ahead anyway, even if it bothers you. An inability to tolerate even discussing sexuality—much less considering how to alter your attitude toward it—may be a big part of what's preventing you from having a fulfilling sex life. Don't let any puritanical gag rule stop you.

A word about sexual orientation: throughout this chapter, I use the pronouns *he* and *she* to refer to the two members of a committed sexual relationship. Most of the issues I discuss, however (such as an imbalance in sex drive between partners, an excessive interest in porn, or recurrent erectile dysfunction) are just as likely to occur in a gay relationship as they are in a straight one. I entreat all my readers—gay and straight—to forgive my sometimes heterocentric shorthand ("she"/"wife"/"girlfriend" rather than "he or she"/"husband or wife"/"girlfriend or boyfriend"), and I urge anyone in a hetero- *or* homosexual relationship to consider that he or she may be on either side of the issue being discussed. Regardless of your gender or sexual orientation, it's possible to have a higher or lower sex drive than your partner, to feel distant from your partner, or to be excessively drawn to porn. The action needed in the relationship remains more or less the same, regardless of the pronouns I'm using. And having your partner—whatever gender—read the section in question can be a jumping-off point for solving the problem for both of you.

Finally, remember to have fun.

It's just sex, after all.

THE SEX AUDIT

1. Do you wish you could have more frequent sex?

2. Do you wish your sexual encounters were more intense and fulfilling?

3. Do you have unrealized sexual fantasies that you have never discussed with your partner?

4. Is your partner no longer sexually attractive to you?

5. Is your partner less interested in sex than in previous months or years?

6. Do you feel your relationship lacks closeness or warmth?

7. Do you interact less frequently with your partner in nonsexual—as well as sexual—ways?

8. Has your use of pornography interfered with your relationship in any way?

9. Do you go to some lengths to hide the frequency of your pornography use?

10. Do you frequently feel too stressed-out or wound-up for sex?

11. Are you frequently despondent or depressed?

12. Are you overweight?

13. Are you on medication for high blood pressure, depression, prostate cancer, or an enlarged prostate?

14. Do you smoke?

15. Do you consume more than six alcoholic drinks a week?

16. Do you take Viagra, Cialis, or any other ED drug?

17. Do you often drink before sex?

18. Do you get less than two hours of intense exercise (running, lifting weights, playing racquet sports), and five hours of mild exercise (walking, swimming, gardening, playing catch) per week?

19. Does your diet lack heart-healthy foods like leafy green vegetables, walnuts, pomegranates, brown rice, and omega-3 fatty acids?

20. Do you have difficulty achieving or maintaining an erection?

"Yes" answers to questions 1–11 suggest that you may have issues with your sex life that are *psychological* in nature.

"Yes" answers to questions 12–19 suggest *physical* problems.

A "Yes" answer to question 20 suggests a problem that could be *physical, psychological,* or *both.*

PSYCHOLOGICAL ISSUES

Issue #1: My Partner Doesn't Want to Have Sex as Much as I Do

In the film *Annie Hall*, Diane Keaton and Woody Allen talk separately to their respective therapists about their sex lives.

"How often do you have sex?" asks Allen's therapist.

"Hardly ever!" he responds. "Three times a week!"

Then Keaton's therapist asks her the same question.

"Constantly," she replies. "Three times a week!"

And therein we have the Big Problem of incompatible sex-drives: one partner (often the man, if it's a male-female relationship) wants sex more often than the other. One feels neglected, the other feels put upon; one feels shut down, the other feels pressured. As funny as the *Annie Hall* scene is, this kind of mismatch can lead to frustration, tension, hostility, and even, finally, to separation and divorce.

Handling the sexual imbalance problem poorly is no laughing matter: MRI research has demonstrated that feeling rejected—as by a partner with lower sex drive in a sex-starved marriage—imprints the brain in the same way that physical pain does.

For men in committed relationships, it's important to remember that women see sex differently from the way we see it. In general—acknowledging that there are exceptions to any blanket statement about either sex—men tend to consider sex in isolation, and women tend to consider sex in context. For men, sex can be mechanical—rub here, push there, squeeze here, and bang, fireworks. For women, the experience is much broader, as much about the environment, what happened during the day, and the bigger picture of what's happening between the two partners as it is about the mechanics of the act itself.

In a scene from the movie *When Harry Met Sally*, Sally describes a sex fantasy in which a faceless hunk rips her clothes off. End of story.

"That's it?" asks Harry, incredulous. "That's the sex fantasy you've been having all these years? And it never changes?"

"Sure it does," she says.

"What's different?"

"What I'm wearing."

Whereas men enjoy pornography—with its zoom-lens focus on penetration—women are considerably more aroused by steamy novels, with their endless descriptions of apparel, setting, and the particular emotional and sexual context of each tension-fraught moment.

So assuming everyone's health is in order (more on that shortly), the over-forty guy whose partner is less receptive than he would like probably needs to *think beyond the bedroom*. Stress, for example, is not conducive to sex for either sex, but women, in particular, have a hard time thinking about sex when they're preoccupied with concerns relating to work or parenting or housekeeping. Some research has even suggested that women have a harder time having sex when there are dirty dishes in the sink!

So if you want more sex, do the dishes. (I'm only half joking.)

"Foreplay," says the renowned sex expert and couples therapist Esther Perel, "should begin immediately after the last time you have sex." That doesn't mean you start kissing or touching right after—it means paying closer attention to her, flirting, teasing, and laughing together more often. It means being attentive to the erotic atmosphere in the relationship at all times—not just in the five minutes right before you have sex.

Couples should ask themselves the following question: *If we met today, would we fall in love with each other?* If the answer is no—if you've let complacency sink into your relationship—you need to put in some time and effort to become the guy your partner fell in love with again. Rediscover the respect, romance, and continual courtship you had in the beginning.

Solution: To improve things in the bedroom, focus on shoring up your relationship outside it.

Issue #2: I Don't Want Sex as Often as My Partner Does

The stereotype would have us believe that in long-term relationships, the husband is always the hard-up initiator and the wife the reluctant responder. But it isn't true. Says the relationship expert Michele Weiner-Davis, "If you think low sexual desire is a women's issue—think again. Low desire in men is one of our very best kept secrets."

Why do we keep this hidden? It comes down to our sense of identity. Men are supposed to be ever ready, always willing, and always able to perform. But we aren't always. No one is.

So what about the times when we just don't want to? What if it seems more trouble than it's worth? (I'm not talking about a mechanical or physiological issue here; I'm talking about a more general *indifference* toward sex: you can achieve an erection, but can take or leave sex—you simply don't feel like it's a big deal).

For your partner's sake, here's the thing to remember: it *is* a big deal. Everyone defines him or herself, in part, through sex. It's a major component in feeling attractive, connected, and loved. It helps men feel masculine and women feel feminine.

Being indifferent to your partner sexually can be devastating, both to her and to the relationship. Lack of sexual intimacy can put you on a slippery slope toward complete disconnection, infidelity, and divorce. And though there are many complex reasons you may lose interest in your partner physically (some of which I'll cover elsewhere in this chapter), there is value—enormous value, sometimes—in making an effort, as an act of kindness to your partner.

There's a good chance you will wind up enjoying it anyway, even if it didn't seem worth the trouble before you began. Though sex proceeds predictably from desire to arousal to orgasm to resolution in most people, the sex researcher and psychiatrist Rosemary Basson has postulated that in some people, arousal *precedes* desire: physical stimulation is a prerequisite for desire to even begin. These are the people who often forget that they enjoy sex until they're in the middle of the act, at which point it becomes intensely pleasurable.

So try just doing it. Put out. Don't wait for the perfect, synchronized timing, the flattering backlight to descend, and for Marvin Gaye to come on the radio. Just dive in, and inspiration will likely follow. As with any aspect of a long-term relationship—finances, parenting, social engagements, housework—your sex life has to be a meeting ground for the needs of both people. If you're the one with the lower sex drive, you may need to recognize that, for your more desirous partner, sex isn't just a mechanical act but an important way to connect and feel appreciated.

Here's a radical idea: if your sex life really needs reigniting, instigate a forty-eight-hour rule: have sex *every forty-eight hours* that you're together, trading off who initiates it each time. It can be any time within that forty-eight-hour window, and it can be any type of sex the initiator wants: fast and dirty, slow and romantic, hot tub, candles, wham-bam-thank-you-ma'am. Doesn't matter. Just carve out time for it every forty-eight hours, regardless of other pressures, and keep it up for thirty days. You'll probably find you want to make it an all-time policy.

Solution: If you have a lower sex drive than your partner, you need to make an effort to step up to the plate now and then, even when you don't think you want to at first.

WHY IS STRAYING SO TEMPTING?

Back in 1995, as you may remember, the actor Hugh Grant was hauled in by the LAPD for hiring a prostitute to give him oral sex in the front seat of his car. You may also remember that Grant was dating Elizabeth Hurley at the time—one of the most beautiful actresses of her era. A couple of weeks after the incident, Jay Leno asked Grant the question that may still be on everyone's mind: *What the hell were you thinking?*

Grant's case is extreme, but his infamous Sunset Boulevard tryst reminds us that regardless of what we've got going on at home, no one is immune from wondering who else is out there.

Why?

Why can't we be happy with what we have—especially when it's someone we love, have chosen to be with, maybe dedicated our lives to and raised children with? Why does the waitress or the coworker or, in Grant's case, the prostitute, turn our heads? And why do our own partners, who may in fact be far better suited to us and even more attractive than these other hypothetical mates, sometimes seem less interesting by comparison?

In other words, what the hell are we thinking?

For the answer, consider a recent study of male rats.

Rats, a species with whom we have more in common than we might like to think, demonstrate an almost endless appetite for novel sex. Science has shown that, when given access to a receptive female, a male rat will copulate enthusiastically at first and eventually lose interest. But when a *new* female rat is introduced, his interest and vigor returns. And the male rat will continue this cycle, doggedly impregnating one female after another like a rodent Genghis Khan, till he literally almost dies.

Scientists call this phenomenon the Coolidge effect, and it happens with humans, too: the frequency and intensity of sex drop off in relationships as time goes by. In their first two years of relationships, 67 percent of gay couples, 45 percent of heterosexual couples, and 33 percent of lesbian couples have sex three times a week or more. For couples who have been together ten years or more, just 11 percent of gay couples, 18 percent of heterosexual couples, and 1 percent of lesbian couples have sex that often. That's a pretty steep drop-off.

Novelty, then, is a huge aphrodisiac, and familiarity breeds . . . if not contempt, exactly, then at least uninterest. *Having*, it turns out, is less erotic than *wanting*. But there's another reason that you, my over-forty friend, and I are particularly vulnerable to the charms and allure of a novel coupling, and that's our old pal T.

Yup, testosterone. You probably remember that, even in healthy men, this essential hormone drops steadily after about age thirty, to the point where many of us begin to feel a serious deficit around midlife. Libido may drop. Energy may wane. Our passion and enthusiasm for life might flag a bit. It's one reason (just one, remember—but an important, biological one) that midlife can start to feel a little black and white as compared with earlier phases of our lives.

What is one of the most reliable ways to boost that flagging T? A new sexual partner. Talk to a guy who has just smart-bombed his whole life to hook up with a new, often younger sexual partner, and he'll tell you it's rejuvenating. Exhilarating. That he feels alive again.

A new sexual partner isn't just about fulfilling one's lusty urges, but about *staying alive*. It's possible that our caveman brains are turned on by the prospect of hooking up with someone who is still capable of bearing children and carrying on our genes—even if our conscious brains have zero interest in being fathers again. And culturally, we associate singleness with vitality, manliness, and the possibility of the thrilling novelty of being with a new partner. Too often we associate couplehood with resignation, irrelevance—even castration ("My wife keeps my balls in a mason jar under the sink.").

So for a guy over forty, the new partner represents another shot at youth, manliness, and immortality. These are indeed powerful and alluring forces. Because as powerful as the promise of sex can be, it's not just sex that's tempting us, but another, more appealing version of ourselves.

Issue #3: The Distance Problem

I feel out of touch with my partner.

Being close to, and friends with, your partner is step one toward ensuring an ongoing, healthy sex life. My wife and I enjoy many activities together: We travel. We exercise. We explore. As I've mentioned, I frequently cook for her—as often as twice a day. To me, she's still a goddess after all these years, and I try to treat her that way. And our strong, mutually respectful friendship—filled with each partner doing kind things for the other on a regular basis—serves as the background for our extremely satisfying sex life.

The poet David Whyte once referred to a good marriage as a "contest of generosity": Which partner can be more attentive to the needs of the other, more receptive to him or her? Does she need a foot massage? Does he need comforting? Does she need you to leave her the hell alone? Do the two of you need a night out together? Do we need a day—or a week—*away* from one another?

If all this sounds challenging, that's because it is. But that's what a fulfilling long-term relationship demands. You won't always get it exactly right; you'll even miss the mark by miles sometimes. And every so often you'll fall into taking one another for granted. It's all okay, as long as you get back up after your screwups and keep trying. At its best, a long-term relationship is akin to surfing or Olympic diving: you have to plunge in, over and over, striving for but never counting on those transcendent moments (in bed or out of it), knowing at every instant you're as likely as not to screw up and take a tumble.

If I were more like many businessmen I know—jetting off all the time and virtually ignoring my wife except when I wanted to have sex—I imagine our sex life would suffer considerably, as it has for most of these men. When you bring the same attention and respect to your long-term relationship that you had when your relationship was new, everybody wins.

That doesn't mean that you'll never have periods where your own desire—or your partner's—diminishes for a while, or when other matters in your life will take priority and the constant romancing will have to be put on hold. We're not bonobos, after all. As with anything in nature, the intensity and passion of your sex life will wax and wane. But a positive, trusting, honest relationship with your partner is one important prerequisite for great sex in the long term.

Solution: Maintain warmth and trust in your relationship with your partner, and trust that although intensity and heat in your sexual relationship may wane for a while, it will return naturally—as long as the two of you maintain your closeness.

WHAT IF I'M TEMPTED?

For most of us, it's not a question of whether you're tempted, but when.

Temptation enters into every long-term relationship. Male or female, straight or gay, we ask an enormous amount of our life partners. She or he is supposed to be our best friend, confidant(e), business partner, collaborator in marriage, and passionate lover to boot. As the sex therapist and author Esther Perel points out, one single person is supposed to provide for all of our basic marriage needs, many of them contradictory: security *and* novelty, predictability *and* adventure, stability *and* risk. And now we live twice as long as we once did.

It's a tall order.

In many movies, these contradictory human needs are symbolized by two different characters, whom a third character—usually a woman—must choose between. In *Shane*, Van Heflin is the hardworking rancher and Alan Ladd is the mysterious gunslinger; in *A Walk on the Moon*, Liev Schrieber is the dependable family man and Viggo Mortensen the rugged bohemian; in *Witness*, Alexander Godunov is the sincere, awkward suitor and Harrison Ford the cowboyish tough guy. Part of what makes these movies effective is that the choice between the two men is inherently impossible: of course, Jean Arthur, Diane Lane, and Kelly McGillis want their life partners to be both reliable and risky.

So do we. We want it *all* from our partners, and we've been sold on the idea that one person can give it to us. All the time.

Is it any wonder, then, that 60 percent of men—and 40 percent of women—cheat on their partners? And this is despite the fact that 91 percent of people say that cheating is among the worst things you can do.

Yet many men in long-term relationships live in denial that they—or their partners—may feel even the remotest stirrings of desire for another person. They feel guilty about any impulses they may experience, and they deny that their partners may ever think about other people. To them, even fantasy is a form of cheating.

Esther Perel calls this kind of thought-policing "intimate terrorism," and I agree. Just because you've committed to someone else doesn't mean that she belongs to you. It's still her choice to be with you, just as it's your choice to be with her. Passion and desire—men's and women's—are never fully knowable, much less tamable. So anyone who is stuck in the antiquated belief that he can fully contain and manage his partner's sexuality is living in a dream world.

So where does that leave us? For men over forty, the extramarital urge is as much a cliché as the steadily growing gut or the ever-receding hairline. What do we do with these urges? Stuff them away, pretend they're not there? Talk them out in therapy, or, more boldly, with one's partner? Or just throw one's existing life away and fully indulge them?

As the sex writer Dan Savage has noted, some gay men seem to have an easier time with this. If one partner is attracted to someone outside the relationship, it's not impossible for both partners to understand that it's very little reflection on them, or on their relationship, it's just something that happens when two vital and sexually active people are out in the world. Many gay couples deal with these situations quite openly, through having a "monogamish" relationship that allows the occasional dalliance (usually within certain parameters), or by role-playing during sex.

Personally, I'm 100 percent in favor of pushing hard to hold on to long-term relationships, and 100 percent not in favor of extramarital affairs. They tend to be messy, drawn-out, and excruciatingly painful for everyone involved. If you're really teetering on the brink of straying, it pays to remember that if you take that plunge, there will come a time when the new person sees you for all your flaws, your annoying personal habits, and your weaknesses, and when you stop seeing her as an obscure object of desire and start seeing her as just another person.

So assuming that you're going to try to keep your marriage intact, step one in dealing with extramarital desire—yours or your partner's—is just to understand that it's completely normal. It may even be an indication that you're both still sexual, that you still have life force coursing through your veins.

Step two is to recognize where your desire is coming from. All affairs are selfish by nature, but what exactly are you seeking in this other person? Attention, validation, excitement? Passion and desire brought on by a situation in which there are roadblocks to sexual consummation? Novelty?

Finally, step three is to ask yourself if you can bring some of the raw material that you or your partner is feeling for the person outside the relationship into your long-term relationship. Instead of looking for those things outside the relationship, can you find them inside it?

The answer, I think, is almost always yes—and the way to do it is to follow the steps in this chapter. If the two of you are always in each other's space, create some distance. Invest time and energy in your passions outside the relationship and apart from one another. Since few obstacles to touching and togetherness exist when two people live together, you may have to create them artificially: decide that you can have any form of intimacy *except* sex for two weeks, or that you'll have sex three times this week—but no nighttime sex, no bedroom sex, and no missionary-position sex. Suddenly you *have* to be creative. And even the buildup to that can be very exciting.

If you've been too distant, on the other hand, carve out time and space to be together. Then, when it comes to sex, get more daring. Understand that, like a garden, sex needs space, air, heat, and feeding to flourish. Much as we guys think "we got the girl, now she's ours forever," this won't happen on its own. Your sexuality, and your partner's, needs care and attention. Flirt, tease, be naughty. Get imaginative. Tell your partner your long-held fantasies and encourage your partner to share hers with you. Then make them happen.

Affairs—and short-term dalliances, one-night stands, and other extramarital sexual adventures—are exceedingly common for men over forty. Because middle age is a time when so many of us feel like we're losing our edge and sliding into mediocrity, the stage is set for a radical lapse of judgment that, for a while anyway, can feel exhilarating.

We still want excitement, to feel alive, to invest our passions in something or someone, to hazard ourselves in the world. Some of us even want those things so desperately we're willing to risk *everything* for them: our marriages, our financial future, our relationships with our children.

Enough guys choose to take that irreversible plunge that I have a hard time condemning them outright for it. But I will say that most of the time, I believe an affair is a bad, bad idea. It's a grab at something that feels real, but it's a misguided one. Often, a guy is seeking something more from what he already has, needing more from his career, marriage, and relationships.

Your New Prime is a time to reinvest in what you already have, to reinfuse it with new life and energy. We all want to be loved, we all want passion, and we all want to feel secure. I believe that a marriage that endures successfully for many decades is one of the more underrated accomplishments in a man's life. Long-term marriage takes boundless passion, endless energy, an abiding curiosity about the other person, and a willingness to reveal and discover yourself, over and over.

Most affairs are a death knell to those things. Women are often perceived as weak if they remain married to a husband who has strayed, so when you get found out (not *if*—you're not as sneaky as you think), the chances are very good that it's all over.

Midlife is an opportunity to choose whether you're going to have a passionate, energetic second act with emotional and physical vitality, or if you're going to throw those things away out of concern for your ego and insecurity. Choose well—this is one you can't take back.

Issue #4: I Support Us—But She Doesn't Want Sex

I make plenty of money and support my partner, while she stays home and takes care of the housework. Still, she's not interested in sex. What's going on?

Having a secure, well-paying job and enough income to support a family is a rarity these days—and certainly something to be proud of. It's also *tough*. Doesn't your partner appreciate all the work you put in? And if so, why is she so indifferent about sex?

Sometimes, like the man says, the problem is you.

It doesn't actually matter that you work hard. Many people are desperate for a job, and some groups, women included, have fought long and hard for the right to work at good jobs. Frankly, I get antsy if I go for too long without putting in a good day's work. That may be happening with your partner, too. As men, we typically define ourselves by our work. Women who don't work may struggle with their sense of identity and self-worth. She may even resent your busy, engaging life outside your relationship. And few of us, male or female, want to have sex when we're feeling lousy about ourselves.

The other thing that may be happening: despite decades of conditioning to the contrary, many hardworking men still assume that, if they're the breadwinner, their wives should handle all the housekeeping, cooking, and child-rearing duties at home. They blithely leave dirty dishes and sweaty underwear wherever they please, assuming that their wife-cum-housekeeper should be more than happy to take care of it (I sincerely hope that's not you).

This assumption is a great way to build hostility and resentment in your relationship even if your partner doesn't work outside the house, and needless to say, it does not make for great sex. Consider: Who washed your dishes and cleaned up your clothes when you were young? If you're like most men, it was your mother. So you're essentially asking your wife or girlfriend to play that role in your relationship.

Sure, now and then it's nice to have someone pick up after you or serve you breakfast in bed. But being "needy"—having a relationship in which one partner regularly takes a parental role toward the other—is doom for sex. Parenting is a great experience, but it isn't sexy. Remember that the next time you expect your wife or girlfriend to pick up your dirty clothes, do all the dishes and laundry, cook all your meals, and then have sex with you. Few women are interested in having sex with a baby who can't take care of himself.

Solution: Help out at home, clean up after yourself, and show appreciation when she does the same for you.

Issue #5: Good Friends—No Heat

My partner and I have a great relationship: connected, warm, supportive. We just don't have sex.

Just as the act of sex requires a buildup of tension before the release of the orgasm, a sexual relationship thrives best when there's tension between the partners—when the air between you crackles, when the mutual desire simmers under the surface, when there's allure, danger, heat. Strip clubs are sexy because the dancers start off clothed. Romantic dinners are sexy because you're gazing into one another's eyes, touching hands, and flirting—but nothing else. The heat builds up, and when you're finally alone together—kids asleep, babysitter paid—the results can be highly combustible.

Here's the irony, though—and the reason I said earlier that a background of intimacy was just step one in assuring an exciting sex life. In some ways, heat can be a distraction in a long-term relationship. When you're trying to raise a family, navigate a challenging career, and manage family finances, you frequently need a spouse who is more of a platonic partner—someone who can help with practical matters and not distract you too much with flashes of skin or lingerie. You need focus and discipline, not electricity and tension.

Thus, long-term relationships built *only* on mutually supportive friendship—while admirable, respectful, and positive—are, by definition, low on tension. The kinks are worked out. "You do the drying, I do the dishes" makes for a clean kitchen—but not necessarily for hot sex. That's why movies and books about passionate relationships usually end before kids and careers—because mutual dependence, practicality, and warmth are, in many ways, curiously *antithetical* to what we consider sexy. As Esther Perel writes in her book *Mating in Captivity*:

> Ironically, what makes for good intimacy does not always make for good sex. It may be counterintuitive, but it's been my experience as a therapist that increased emotional intimacy is often accompanied by decreased sexual desire. This is indeed a puzzling inverse correlation: the breakdown of desire appears to be an unintentional consequence of the creation of intimacy.

So where does that leave us? Being good friends—maybe best friends—with the person you live with is part of what makes day-to-day life rewarding and fulfilling. For example, my wife, Maria, and I are best friends with a long history. We have shared the parenting load together for nearly a quarter century, and along the way we have had to work through conflicts and compromises, and otherwise tend to the thousand practical details of day-to-day living, very few of which could possibly be construed as sexy.

So I'm definitely *not* saying "Don't have a positive and workable day-to-day relationship with your partner." Far from it; remember, that's step one. I'm just saying that for some people, this kind of stable relationship can run at cross-purposes with having an exciting sex life, and many people find that these two apparently contradictory desires—the one for stability and comfort and the other for adventure and novelty—are impossible to reconcile in one relationship. Hence the time-honored stereotype of men marrying a "respectable" woman to raise the kids while keeping a wilder, more sexually adventurous woman as a mistress.

Short of that highly compromised and potentially disastrous setup, though, what can New Primers in long-term relationships do to continue to want what we already have? Are we doomed to cheat on our partners, become porn addicts, or simply be unhappy and unfulfilled in our sex lives now and forever?

Absolutely not.

I submit that teenage groping isn't *just* exciting because young hormones are raging, but because of the planning, the danger of getting caught, and the buildup. If you were lucky enough to have a partner in high school, you spent most of your time wondering how and when you were going to hook up. You planned. You fantasized. You wondered how she would look, what she might say, and what you might say in response. Your hookup sessions, however tame or hot they got by your standards now, had significance: you were fully engaged, mind, body, spirit, imagination.

In a long-term relationship, you're lucky to get two minds and two bodies in the same room at once. Sex is often rote and repetitious.

The solution, paradoxically, is to find a way to bring more mystery, more charge, and more tension into the sexual component of your relationship, amid the low-tension, low-charge background you create through normal day-to-day closeness and intimacy. That may mean planning for sex, prolonging the buildup, and making it into something of an event again, just as you did when you were younger. Checking into a hotel for a night, meeting for drinks after work, even having a date in which you pretend you've never met before (like Phil and Claire on *Modern Family*) can lead to the feeling of novelty and discovery that leads to great sex.

It may also very well mean giving your partner more space and distance, which then allows desire to grow.

What does that mean?

In addition to all the things you do together, do the two of you also have separate interests, pursuits, and passions? As long as you have a strong foundation of love and trust in the relationship, a certain amount of distance and difference is ultimately good for a relationship—particularly for the sexual aspect of a relationship. Distance breeds desire no less now than it did when you were a teenager; you need to know that a person is *separate* from you in order to feel *attracted* to her in turn. Consider that the best sex you have with a long-term partner tends to be makeup sex, reunion sex, or sex after a stress-induced layoff—sex that follows a period of deprivation during which you're reminded that your partner is *different* from you. Distance allows your imagination to run wild, and your fantasy life has room enough to become fertile again.

Solution: Cultivating some novelty and mystery in your relationship—against the backdrop of closeness—is essential for an exciting sex life. Give your partner space for her own interests and passions, take space for yours in your own life, and allow sexual anticipation and heat to grow.

THE RELATIONSHIP REBOOT

A funny thing happened while I was researching and writing about the topic of optimizing a long-term relationship and improving your sex life: I moved out of the house.

When I say those words, most people are aghast. They assume that my quarter-century-plus marriage is on the rocks, that one or both of us must have been unfaithful, and that Maria and I must be on the fast track to divorce.

None of it's true. Instead, we're doing what I'm calling a Relationship Reboot. And I think it's the best thing we've done for our marriage in a long time.

After twenty-seven years of marriage (and thirty-five years' being together), we both realized we had lost a lot of the spontaneity, energy, and passion that was so abundant in our earlier life. After collaborating as parents and partners in running both the household and our companies, we had become more like business partners than passionate husband and wife.

We've seen many, many couples break up for this very reason over the years. Newport Beach, California, where I currently live and work, must be the divorce capital of the world. A functional couple with more than ten years of marriage behind them is a huge anomaly, and one with over twenty is rare indeed.

So instead of letting our relationship spiral further downward, we decided to do a Relationship Reboot.

Here's how we're doing it: I moved to a nice-but-modest apartment a mile from our house. All that's there is a bed, a yoga mat, and a meditation cushion. My wife is staying in our house, but she has a key and access to my place. We're deeply immersed in our own lives—me in my business ventures and the writing of this book, she in managing the house, our kids, and the operation of our companies. Once or twice a week, we go out on a date, work out together, or spend time at our house, where I cook us dinner. Knowing that the time is special, we have a great evening together, focusing completely on one another, the way we did before kids, job pressures, and other distractions became the reality of our life together. At the end of most of these evenings, we have great sex, though it's not a foregone conclusion. And then I head back to my monk-like apartment until our next date. Some nights she sneaks out of the house for a late-night rendezvous, which we plan with anticipation (and hide from our kids as if they were the parents!).

We have a few ground rules:

- This isn't a "hall pass" for either one of us. We aren't looking to hook up with anyone else.

- When we get together, it's for real dates. We dress up and do something special and unique, not just hang out in sweats at the house or go to the movies.

- Importantly, we behave in all other respects as if we were at the beginning of our relationship: surprise gifts, spontaneous texts, romantic phone calls. No complacency or expectations. We're courting and dating again—trying to "win" the other person by showering her or him with attention and thoughtfulness.

I have every intention of moving back in. Our plan is to time it for when our second daughter leaves for college in a few months. What we're doing, very consciously, is creating an obstacle to intimacy to allow our desire to grow again. To see one another as separate people again. To reacquaint ourselves with who we are outside this thirty-five-year partnership—and with whom we fell in love.

In all honesty, one of our problems was too much sex. Passion ran high (as I've stated, my T levels run abnormally high), and we had a great sex life. But like everything else, if you have too much of a good thing, you start to take it for granted. When every day is special, no day is.

Sex is a key component to a great relationship, but it's definitely not all there is to it—as anyone in a long-term partnership can attest. It's necessary, but not sufficient. A sports entrepreneur I know used to regale me each time I saw him with tales of having had twice-daily sex with his wife of seventeen years every day since they married. Despite all that, he still had an affair—and his marriage ended in a nasty divorce.

To take my marriage to the next level, and to restore real passion and intimacy, I had to see my way to the very un-guy-ish realization that just because the sex is frequent and satisfying, it does not mean that a marriage is all it can be. And that's one of the reasons we decided on a reboot.

Is it for you? Maybe, maybe not. I realize it's a stretch logistically and financially for most. But there are many different setups for a satisfying partnership, with the long-term, monogamous cohabitation that's widely accepted as "correct" in our society being just one of many. Some people sleep in separate beds. Others (famously, Kurt Russell and Goldie Hawn) sleep in separate houses on the same property. Maria and I decided on a period of planned separation to stave off complacency and get back the spark, intimacy, and passion we had when we met all those years ago.

For us, it's working brilliantly and has taken our marriage and sex life to the next level. And if you can get past the raised eyebrows, it may work for you as well.

Issue #6: Unfulfilled Fantasies

I have an active fantasy life when it comes to sex, but my actual sex life with my partner is dull.

I believe "safe sex"—default, missionary, day-to-day, nothing-new sex—grows out of our desire for normalcy and predictability. It's not challenging for either partner; you don't have to think about it; it does what it's supposed to do. It's like your favorite easy-to-cook meal: it fills you up, it's satisfying, it's convenient, but not much else. It's forgotten almost as soon as it's over.

Great sex, like a great meal, needs more attention, more preparation, and more forethought than the run-of-the-mill variety, and if that sounds like more work to you, remember all the work you used to have to put in to arrange those super-intense grope sessions with your high school sweetheart. Amazing sex in Your New Prime requires at least that much attention and planning.

I can't (and won't, don't worry) give you instructions on exactly what to do once you're alone together. But I will say that the best sex isn't tame. It's not predictable or socially acceptable. It's not—to quote Esther Perel—"politically correct." You may want something that your partner thinks is completely whacko—and she may want the same from you as well. The best sex pushes boundaries, even (maybe especially) when a couple has been together a long time. Push the boundaries of who you think you're supposed to be and who your partner is supposed to be and you're suddenly in new territory; you automatically inject some of the danger into the sexual relationship that you found when you were first discovering sex as a younger man.

Even with all the experience we over-forty men have had over the years, and even with sexual images in our faces all the time, shame and embarrassment remain potent forces in our bedroom behavior. It makes sense, because for most of us, our sexual tastes and fantasies are inextricably linked with our deepest fears and vulnerabilities—and to expose them is to expose ourselves to ridicule and rejection. That's why it's so easy to go just for meat-and-potatoes sex, even when fantasizing about the caviar-and-truffles variety; it's hard to ask for something off the beaten path without worrying whether your partner will respond with enthusiasm, disgust, or horror.

On the other hand, busting through all those layers of repression and asking for what you want can be incredibly liberating and gratifying, and I have no doubt that your partner will respond positively to it. She may not be entirely up for everything you suggest, but in all likelihood she has unexpressed, unrealized fantasies she'd like to explore as well, and by opening up about yours, you encourage a much more meaningful sexual connection. Yes, it may feel weird or edgy or dangerous at first, but being on your edge is exactly what makes for the best sex.

Since the days of Kinsey, the idea of what constitutes "normal" sexual behavior has expanded to include virtually anything legal to which both parties consent. So if your thing is dressing up, or role-playing, or taking pictures, or driving her crazy with a vibrator, or tying one another up and spanking the daylights out of each other . . . knock yourself out. It's all fair game, and it might well be just what the other person secretly desires.

Solution: Life's short. Be willing to ask for what you want in the bedroom—in a tactful and undemanding way—and to do what your partner wants as well.

Issue #7: Passion, Lost and Found

Even though we try, my partner and I don't turn each other on.

For all our sophistication and intellect, we can't escape the fact that, sexually speaking, we're animals, driven as much by instinct as by intellect. We look at one person and find her or him instantly attractive. We look at someone else and . . . *meh*. She may be the most objectively beautiful person in the world and still not turn you on. Our taste is what it is—no faking.

In a way, that should be good news: whether you're heavy, thin, muscular, tall, short, you can still find someone who's attracted to you. But from another perspective, it can be distressing: is there nothing to be done if my partner isn't interested in me anymore?

There absolutely is.

The solution is to reconnect to your animal self. And that's easier than you think.

As an aphrodisiac, exercise is underrated. Physiologically speaking, it's far sexier than smoking, drinking, drugs, sleepless nights, and sax solos that get all the credit for being perfect mood-setters. For one thing, exercise boosts blood flow and self-esteem while heightening physical sensation and improving confidence and body image. And it's our confidence and body image that may well be more important to how we're perceived than our body type or the number on the scale.

One recent study also found that when heterosexual strangers were placed together in situations that spiked adrenaline (as exercise does), mutual sexual attraction increased. Exercising together—as I often do with Maria—can be competitive, playful, and very sensual. Being physical with one another in this nonsexual context gives you the opportunity to appreciate and admire one another's bodies from a distance. That look-but-don't-touch vibe can be very charged. And exercising together in the morning, when T levels naturally peak, may be even better because it combines a hormonally charged environment with the confidence boost both of you get from working out. Overall, working out regularly—by yourself or with your partner—is a great way to pave the road for more intimate forms of movement.

In a larger sense, taking good care of your body is also a good way to take care of your partner: it keeps you looking and feeling young, healthy, virile, and vigorous, making you more attractive to her. Your energy, mood, and mental capacities also improve, which makes you better company. In general, women appreciate men who take care of themselves, just as men appreciate partners who put in the time and energy necessary to look good for them. Many women think nothing of spending at least an hour a day on exercise and another half hour to an hour on their hair, skin, and nails so they can look radiant, healthy, and beautiful. As women get older, they often spend more time and energy on looking and feeling their best. Men usually spend less. Remember that next time you stumble out of the house looking unshaven, uncombed, and exhausted.

So exercise (following the recommendations in chapter 4) and good physical care are obvious ways to keep yourself attractive and spark a physical attraction from your partner, while improving sexual functioning at the same time. It's a no-brainer.

Solution: To stoke the passion fires, do other enjoyable physical (but nonsexual) activities together.

Issue #8: Exercise Killed My Sex Life

I work out all the time, but it's doing nothing for my sex life. In fact, it seems to be getting worse.

A word of caution for exercise fiends: too much exercise may push your sex drive in the wrong direction.

How? By overstressing your autonomic nervous system.

Here's a quick physiology lesson: your autonomic nervous system operates on a continuum between two major settings. On one end of the spectrum, there's the *sympathetic* side, which clicks on when you fight, flee, or freeze; on the other, there's the *parasympathetic* side, which kicks in when you need to rest, digest, recuperate, or reproduce. The former, a high-stress setting, is *catabolic*: you burn calories, break down muscle tissue, and get ready for a literal or figurative war. The latter, a low-stress setting, is *anabolic*: you're rebuilding damaged muscle tissue, or kicking back after a long day, a hard workout, or a big meal.

Most of the time, the autonomic nervous system works in a seesaw fashion: as the "ramp-up" sympathetic side turns on, the "cool-down" parasympathetic side turns off. We toggle easily between the two extremes—revving up into a sympathetic state when we work out hard, confront the boss, or meet a prospective client, then chilling back out to the parasympathetic side after we get home from work, hug our kids, and have a nice meal.

However, when stress gets too overwhelming, our autonomic nervous system can get stuck on the "stressed-out and harried" setting. This is part of why it's virtually impossible to get busy in the bedroom when you're too busy out of it: you end up stuck in sympathetic overdrive, so your body, biologically, wants no part of rest, relaxation, or reproducing. Instead, it's afraid for its life. Because of this, we wind up feeling god-awful much of the time: run-down, frayed, nauseated, and turned off.

Generally speaking, exercise is a powerful balancer of the autonomic nervous system—first it revs you up, then it leaves you feeling calmer and more centered. Too much exercise, however, may have the opposite effect. Exercise, after all, is a stressor—much like a major undertaking at work or an argument with a family member—and if you're overtrained, burned-out, and unable to recover from one workout to the next, your body remains in a catabolic state that kills libido.

So if you're a compulsive exerciser, working out for many, many hours per week in hopes of developing the perfect physique, you may find that your desire and performance in the bedroom take a distressing nosedive. There's also a possibility that your exercise habits have tipped over into narcissism, and that your partner's starting to sense that you're lavishing too much attention on your own curves and not enough on hers. Either way, the solution is to back way off for a week or two, do some enjoyable, low-stress activities together for exercise, and return to your workouts only after you feel ready. This should be when your sleep habits, appetite, and sexual desire have returned to normal, your energy is high, and your mental attitude is on track.

Yoga may be your best bet for an exercise option during this time: the ancient practice has been shown to improve sexual functioning in both men and women. A 2010 study of sixty-five men, aged twenty-four to sixty, found that twelve weeks of yoga improved every aspect measured of sexual functioning, intercourse satisfaction, performance, confidence, partner sychronization, erection, ejaculatory control, and orgasm. A concurrent study of women aged twenty-five to fifty-five had similar results: measures of desire, arousal, lubrication, orgasm, satisfaction, and pain all improved following the twelve-week yoga intervention.

Solution: Dial down on the intense workouts for a while, and de-stress with some yoga—ideally with your partner.

Issue #9: A Porny Dilemma

I'm more into porn than I am into my partner.

Back when we were kids, catching sight of a naked breast—even a *photograph* of a naked breast—was a complex operation that required near-military levels of planning and execution.

First, you had to know someone who had access—usually someone's older brother. Maybe someone told you he had some hot topless pics. Then you had to get in good with the appropriate parties, which might have involved a cash exchange. Next you had to make it happen—show up at the right place, at the right time, when no one's parents were around, to catch a glimpse of a dog-eared shot of Miss November 1975 in candy-striper shorts and a strategically misplaced feather boa. It was the best seventeen seconds of your young teenage life.

Things are a little different now.

Today, porn is *everywhere*. Mistype a letter or two of your favorite website and there's a good chance you'll wind up taking in a lot more action than the latest sports highlights.

A few mind-blowing stats on Internet porn:

- An estimated 30 percent of all bandwidth on the Internet is porn.

- Porn sites have 450 million unique visitors every month—more than Netflix, Amazon, and Twitter *combined.*

- Sixty-seven percent of men ages thirty-one to forty-nine view porn at least monthly.

- Two-thirds of professionals have porn on their work computers.

- The bandwidth for YouPorn.com, a popular porn hub, is six times larger than what's needed for Hulu.com.

Who watches porn? Everyone. Married, unmarried, gay, straight, male, and yes, even female. The puritanical set can rail against it all they want, but something that popular and that satisfying to a basic human need will never want for an audience. And I'll bet the farm that anyone who vocally disapproves is watching it anyway, probably as you read these very words. So if you harbor any guilt whatsoever about your porn habits, whatever they may entail, it's time to get over it.

In case you haven't discovered the joys of Internet porn just yet, by all means, jump on the Web and have at it. I'll see you back here in twelve minutes (the average length of a visit to a porn site).

I'd like to submit that, contrary to what your mother or your priest or the uptight girl-friend you had in 1983 may have told you, I believe it's okay to use porn periodically (and I stress *periodically*). It may even be healthy. One 2007 study of six hundred Danish men and women reported that porn had an overall positive effect on "sexual knowledge, attitudes toward sex, attitudes towards and perception of the opposite sex, sex life and general quality of life." Contradicting a long-held assumption about the effects of porn, a 2009 study from the University of Montreal found that men who watched porn did not find that it changed their views of women or affected their relationships.

Most compelling of all is a 2010 study that found that, concurrent with an increased availability of pornography in Denmark, "there was a significant *decrease* in the number of sex offenses registered by the police in Copenhagen. . . . Various factors suggest that the availability of pornography was the direct cause of this decrease" (italics mine). Contrary to the conservative views on "smut," then, porn can be seen as much more of a safety valve than a fuse for deviant and damaging sexual behavior.

In spite of what you may have heard, most men are able to distinguish between the real world and the porn-fantasy world, just as they are able to distinguish between the real world and the action-movie world or the video-game world. Men know it's a fantasy world—it's just one they like to visit now and then.

So is porn 100 percent harmless then?

Unfortunately, no. Though porn has been around for thousands of years (in 2005, archaeologists in Germany reported finding an artist's depiction of a copulating couple that was 7,200 years old), the recent accessibility of porn—along with its recent acceptability—offers a new set of potential pitfalls for men not unlike the problems that arose with junk food.

Consider: as humans, our main drives are, first, surviving, and, second, passing on our genes. Back when we were hunter-gatherers, it was beneficial to gorge ourselves whenever delicious, palatable food was available, because the food might go bad soon and we never knew when we'd get to eat again.

Similarly, when and if the opportunity to have lots of sex with many different partners ever came up, our ability to perform was beneficial for the survival of our species, as such a sex jackpot would have been a rare opportunity to spread our genes as widely as possible in a short amount of time. Even a knuckle-dragging caveman knew that.

Until very recently, then, there was no upside to having an off switch for our desire for novel sexual situations—just as there was no upside to having an off switch for our desire for sweet foods. For our ancient ancestors, it was better to binge on palatable food, and willing sexual partners, while the bingeing was good.

Remember those lucky male rats and their endless stream of willing-and-able female companions? No matter how hot the rat-on-rat sex was at first, eventually the male lost interest. But when a new female rat was introduced, it was game on all over again.

Like those oversexed male rats, we, too, are hardwired for novelty. Old partners lose their appeal and new partners turn us on. We can't help it—it's an animal response. Now, we can certainly override that response by making considered choices that are good for our relationships in the long term, just as we can override our homicidal impulses toward the guy who cuts us off on the freeway. But that doesn't mean those impulses aren't there. And it's probably healthier to indulge those impulses in a harmless way than to deny that they exist altogether.

Internet porn, it turns out, is especially well suited to provide the illusion of precisely the kind of novelty our caveman brains crave. Don't like the blonde with the cowboy hat? Click on the brunette in the nurse's uniform. Lose interest in her? Try the site with the cartoon Japanese coeds. As with fast-food restaurants, soda machines, and the snack food aisle in convenience stores, the system is set up almost perfectly to create, and then cater to, our addictions.

And as it turns out, *addiction* isn't too strong a word for some of us. Science is demonstrating that, for addicts, the substance or behavior in question matters less than the response of the brain's pleasure-reward system to that substance or behavior. And too much Internet porn, just like too much gambling or shopping or cheesecake, dampens the dopamine response in the brain—which in turn makes us crave more (or kinkier versions) of it. This sets up a cycle of addiction that closely resembles what you see in alcoholics and drug addicts.

Among users of porn, "porn-induced erectile dysfunction" is, unsurprisingly, an increasing problem. Overly frequent masturbation to extreme imagery can lead you to become desensitized to the sights, sounds, and sensations of real sex, and it can inhibit your sexual performance right when you need it most.

So though I'm agnostic on the morality of porn—and even somewhat relieved that porn use doesn't carry the stigma that it once did—it can become a serious problem, particularly in the technologically enhanced form that most guys are consuming it these days.

Now that we have 24-7 access to Miss November and to all forms of high-def video flesh, what are we to do? How do we tell the difference between moderate use and a serious problem?

I may be a Luddite in this regard, but I think that, in general, men need to monitor their use of technology as a stand-in for social interaction of all kinds, including (perhaps especially) sexual interaction. We're social animals, after all, and though electronic inter-action has its uses, it will never stand in for face-to-face and body-to-body interaction any more than Mountain Dew should replace spring water or Apple Jacks should replace ap-ples. The ersatz stuff should never replace the real stuff that we evolved to thrive on. In the same way, porn should never replace your relationship with an actual, physical partner. If you're in a long-term relationship, porn shouldn't be a substitute for connecting—sexually or otherwise—with your partner; if you're single, porn shouldn't become your girlfriend (think Joaquin Phoenix in *Her*), or prevent you from dating or connecting with eligible partners. I believe that over time, excessive porn use can desensitize you to the nuances of real relation-ships. Porn works best as a temporary placeholder, a way of scratching an itch, not a way of giving meaning to your life.

According to the experts, the frequency of your porn use is less important than its effect on the rest of your life. If you think you may have a problem, consider the following questions:

1. Have you seen an uptick in your use of porn? This could mean using it more frequently, but it could also mean needing kinkier or more shocking forms of porn to become aroused.

2. Have you been investing more time, money, or energy to obtain or use porn? That is, has porn started to infringe on other areas of your life? Do you use porn when you should be working, studying, or spending time with your kids?

3. Has porn created a rift in your relationships? Has it affected your sex life or other aspects of your relationship? Are you less able to become aroused without porn? Have you been caught using porn at work? Has it become something you go to great lengths to hide?

If the answer to any or all of these questions is yes, take a porn fast. That's right: no porn and no masturbation (!) for two weeks. If that seems like forever, you may need to enlist the help of a support group (recovery.org or sexualrecovery.com are good places to start). But the period of abstinence will give your pleasure centers time to reboot. Afterward, you should go back to regular sex (assuming you're with a partner), and masturbate the old-fashioned way: using your old mental warehouse of sexual memories and images (a.k.a. your "BOMB": Beat-Off Memory Bank).

Which might even include that dog-eared shot of Miss November.

STOKING THE FIRES:
SEVEN THINGS EVERY RELATIONSHIP NEEDS

There's a deluge of relationship advice out there: books, articles, lectures, certifications, retreats, movies, professional opinions, and more (and I'm only adding to it all—sorry). As with any topic, some of what you hear is beneficial, some is decidedly not, and plenty of it is just noise.

In an effort to help you see the forest for the trees in the thorny thicket of relationship advice, here are seven key elements of keeping passion alive in a long-term relationship:

1. COMMUNICATION

You know those sounds that come out of your partner's mouth on a regular basis? Those are *words*. Words are important. Communication is the sine qua non of a good relationship: nail this one element and the rest is likely to fall into place. But if you aren't connecting, talking, and processing together on a regular basis, you're on autopilot, friend. Time to grab the ball and go deep—just like you used to.

2. QUALITY TIME

Just because you're in the same room—even the same bed—doesn't mean you're actually connecting to one another. Plenty of guys I know are so absorbed in their work and so distracted by their children that they barely utter a word to their wives all day that doesn't have to do with logistics of paying the bills or picking up the kids. Most of your time together may not be quality time. So don't be the guy who wakes up after twenty-five years of marriage and realizes he no longer knows his wife.

3. TIME TO YOURSELF

A smart older guy I once knew, with a half century of marriage under his belt, described a good marriage as a three-part dance: the man's dance alone, the woman's dance alone, and their dance together. Too much time together can become too much time together. You both need a few separate interests, friends, and pursuits in order to bring something novel into the relationship. Time apart is nourishing and heats things up when you get back together. Take it for yourself, and make her take it too. And know that any extra time you spend with your kids solo will not be time you regret.

4. SHOW AND TELL

The relationship expert Dr. Gary Chapman has identified five ways to express love: affirming words, giving gifts, spending quality time, performing acts of service, and touching physically. You don't necessarily need to hit them all, and your partner is likely to respond more to some than others. Figure out which ones they are, and double down on them when you do.

5. APPRECIATION

A writer friend of mine has a girlfriend who brings him snacks and drinks throughout his day at his desk. She drops these things off without a word, and in the moment, he doesn't thank her.

Later on, though, he's enormously demonstrative with his appreciation. He knows that without those little deliveries of sustenance, his day wouldn't be nearly as productive. But he also knows that for his own process, if he took even a moment to interrupt his focus to thank her—much less give her a hug and ask about her day—it would take him much longer to get back into the flow of writing.

At other times, he's the one doting on her. She's a dancer, so he's the one at the studio space setting up all afternoon before the show, helping to put everything away afterward, and showering her with flowers for all her efforts. Both partners sacrifice for one another at different times and in different ways.

The point: appreciate your partner for who she is and what she does whenever and however you can. Accept that sometimes you'll be the appreciator, and sometimes the apprecia-tee.

6. SEX

This is key, foundational, and fundamental. If you're not having sex, even if both of you are willing and able, that makes you roommates, just like you had in college. Is that the type of relationship you want with your life partner?

You can only fool yourself for so long that you're just fine without all the bother . . . and the same goes for her. You need each other, so find a way to make it happen.

7. NOVELTY

This means finding ways to remain curious about your partner emotionally, intellectually, and sexually. In the same way that you are evolving (your needs aren't the same as they were twenty years ago), so is she. In the same way that you don't always know what you need or want now as opposed to twenty years ago, neither does she. So figure it out together. Challenge one another. Ask tough questions, and give real answers.

PHYSICAL ISSUES

So far, most of this chapter has been about the psychological and relational aspects of sexual performance. That's by design: the physical state of your plumbing is only one factor, and probably not the most important one, in determining the state of your sex life.

Still, as we approach our middle years, many of us begin to experience erectile dysfunction that *does* have a physical basis—and it can be extremely frustrating for everyone, perhaps ourselves most of all. Back in the day, a flash of toned, tanned female skin could make us horny for hours; now that we're older, it seems that only a three-hour visit to a Persian pleasure dome will get the slightest rise out of us—which can be terribly disconcerting. Because one of my companies sells products to improve men's health, I sometimes receive phone calls from complete strangers who are in a genuine panic about their declining sexual performance. I get it: sexual functioning represents a fundamental part of who we are as men. It's sad that so few of us feel comfortable talking about these issues—the physical and the psychological ones—with anyone close to us.

There are tons of interventions out there for ED—some psychological, some medical, some complete nonsense. But before you pop any pills or undergo surgery, make sure you've tried adjusting your lifestyle first.

One major point I'd like to hammer home here is that when it comes to your health, everything is connected. You can't skimp on sleep or eat a lousy diet or skip exercise for long without something going wrong somewhere. Maybe that something will be chronic back pain, depression, or headaches. Maybe it will be ED. Regardless, you can't get away with poor health habits for long. Here are a few of the worst offenders (some of which will be familiar at this point), along with tips for improvement:

Issue #1: You Eat a Crappy Diet

The same stuff that causes your belly to grow causes your penis to shrink. Simple sugars, foods rich in inflammatory omega-6 fats, processed foods, and fried foods can all contribute to decreased circulation—and therefore to erectile dysfunction as well. Conversely, diets rich in fruits, vegetables, whole grains, heart-healthy fats, and fish tend to improve sexual functioning.

A few additional dietary hard-on boosters to try:

- chilis
- bananas
- salmon
- pork
- cherries
- onions
- wine
- oats
- beets

Issue #2: You Need a Boost

Sometimes potency problems crop up because you're not getting enough of something in your diet. Vitamins and naturopathic remedies can be particularly helpful when you're stressed and not eating or sleeping well as a result. The supplements below—many of them covered in chapter 1—can all improve erectile functioning, including:

- L-arginine
- Pygeum africanum
- plant sterols
- Trubulus terrestris
- fenugreek
- vitamin D3
- Avena sativa

- L-citrulline
- green tea
- beet root
- Ginkgo biloba
- Resveratrol
- acetyl L-carnitine

All these ingredients can be found in their proper dosages and ratios in my doctor-approved EveryDay Male formula from PR Labs—a supplement I take daily and wholeheartedly endorse.

Issue #3: You're Carrying Extra Weight

Ever notice how hard your car has to work when your trunk is loaded with luggage, sandbags, or barbell weights? That's how hard your heart has to work when you're carrying a lot of extra weight around your middle. Extra pounds are inherently tough on the heart, and thus on your sexual performance. Type 2 diabetes, which can result from weight gain, can in turn damage the nerves that supply the penis, resulting in ED. Lose the LBs through the smart diet and exercise techniques described in this book, and your functioning will improve.

Exercising will also help increase blood flow, improve cardiovascular health, increase testosterone, and improve self-image—all of which can contribute positively to better sexual functioning. No matter who you are, you can't afford not to be exercising.

Issue #4: You Have High Blood Pressure (or High Cholesterol)

As I mentioned in the nutrition chapter, erectile dysfunction is a powerful indicator of cardiovascular problems: 75 percent of men with heart disease also have problems achieving an erection. Consider recurring ED as a warning sign that you need to adopt heart-healthy behaviors. It's survival of the firmest.

Your blood vessels constantly have blood flowing through them and are under some strain all the time. But when your blood pressure and cholesterol are high, they're particularly at risk—and that includes the vessels that supply blood to your penis. If you are prone to high cholesterol, make sure you monitor it at every doctor's visit, and check your blood pressure frequently. If you don't own a good blood pressure cuff, many drugstores offer checks for free.

Ironically, blood pressure drugs, such as hydrochlorothiazide, spironolactone, and beta-blockers like Atenolol may actually cause ED, which is another reason to work on lowering your BP the old-fashioned way through diet and exercise, rather than with drugs.

Issue #5: You're a Chimney

If you're a smoker, you don't need me to tell you to stop. But hey: *Stop.* For real. It isn't just your heart and lungs that are paying the price. Smoking also damages arteries, doubling your risk of ED.

Even if full cessation isn't in the cards in your immediate future, at least take a day off when there's a good chance of fireworks in bed in the next twenty-four hours. One recent study suggested that impotent smokers can see a 40 percent improvement in ED symptoms after just one day without puffing.

Issue #6: You're Too Hardwired

I've already sounded off about porn quite a bit in this chapter, but porn-induced erectile dys-function is a real condition. Just as Pavlov could condition his dogs to salivate at the sound of a bell, using too much porn can teach you that the time to stand at attention is when you power up your laptop, rather than when your partner gives you that come-hither look (in the porn-addiction comedy *Don John*, the protagonist gets turned on when he hears the boot-up chord on his Apple computer). Porn can also lead indirectly to self-image issues and performance anxiety: *Can I go at it like a jackrabbit for forty-five minutes straight like the guy in the porn flicks? Is that what she wants?* If you're a frequent and enthusiastic porn user who is having trouble connecting with a real partner, time to power off and focus on reality for a while.

Issue #7: You're Stressed-Out

Achieving an erection is a function of the parasympathetic nervous system; that's why you need to be relaxed before you can pull one off. If your sympathetic nervous system is working overtime due to stress and anxiety, you just won't be able to stand at attention. And that may lead to a vicious cycle of more anxiety and stress—which in turn can make an erection even more difficult to maintain.

De-stressing is sometimes a big-picture life problem: you need to scale back on work, sort through some difficulties in your relationships, maybe even change careers. In an acute phase of stress, deep breathing, meditation, massage, and other stress-reduction techniques can be a huge help—and in fact should be a regular part of your routine.

Just focusing on each of your senses, one at a time, can have an immediate calming effect. You don't even need to stop what you're doing. Driving to work, you can focus on the smell of your car seats, the feel of the steering wheel, and the sight of the sunlight on the trees. Washing dishes, you can focus on the feel of the water and soap, the weight of the dish you're washing, the light reflecting through the stream of water in the sink. Do that for three minutes and you'll detect a noticeable difference in your anxiety and stress levels.

Issue #8: Your T is on E

Though it's not a direct link, there is a correlation between low testosterone and ED. T in the normal to high range boosts mood, confidence, and sex drive, all of which can improve sexual performance. And low T is a symptom of several health problems—diabetes and obesity among them—that in turn cause ED. You also need some T to achieve an erection at all: no T, no E.

So if your T levels are flagging, boost them up using some of the natural techniques in chapter 1. At worst, you'll decrease your belly fat, increase your insulin sensitivity (your capacity to digest carbs), and lower your risk for diabetes and obesity—all of which will help your member man up.

Issue #9: You Need a Good Poke

Acupuncture—the ancient practice of painlessly inserting tiny needles just under the skin along various "meridian lines" of the body—can be remarkably effective at reversing psychologically rooted ED. Sixty-four percent of men who underwent acupuncture treatments were symptom-free after six weeks. And in case you're worrying—the needles go in your *back*.

Issue #10: You Commonly Have One (or Seven) Too Many

In moderation, alcohol has little effect on potency. But too much, as Shakespeare said, "provokes the desire, but it takes away the performance." Blood flow to the penis is reduced, as is the intensity of orgasm. Short-term, the result is that alcohol inhibits most men's capacity to achieve and maintain an erection, and some men are unable to have an erection at all after drinking. Long-term, 60 to 70 percent of heavy drinkers experience sexual problems, including ED. Solution? Ease up on the sauce.

Issue #11: Your Toxin Load Is Too High

BPA and phthalates—both ubiquitous chemicals found in plastics of all kinds, including those used to store food—may have serious effects on male sexual performance. One 2010 Kaiser Permanente study found that men with elevated BPA in their urine were more likely to experience worsening male sexual functioning, including ED and reduced libido, than men with lower levels. Phthalates have been found to disrupt the synthesis of testosterone, a hormone that is vital to maintaining a healthy libido.

Avoid these erection-deflators by eating fresh and organic fruits, vegetables, grains, and meats; eating at home as much as possible; avoiding canned foods and all cups and bottles with BPA (recycling numbers 1, 2, 4, or 5 on the container means it's BPA-free; avoid 3, 6, and 7); using a stainless steel bottle for drinking water instead of a plastic one; and storing food in glass containers (for more on toxins, see chapter 1).

ANOTHER REASON TO HAVE MORE SEX: YOUR PENIS NEEDS THE EXERCISE!

All healthy men with normal erectile function have multiple nighttime erections during their sleep cycle—and not just because we're dreaming about Alessandra Ambrosio. Nocturnal erections serve several purposes: they promote oxygenation and blood flow in the penis, which help prevent ED; from a biological perspective, assuming a partner is nearby, they encourage reproduction; and they also help to maintain penis size by repeatedly stretching the penile tissue.

Little did you know that while you were sleeping, your little friend was pumping up and down so that you could perform better when called on for action!

As you age, however, nocturnal erections become less frequent and less stiff—mostly due to decreased testosterone—and you lose out on these benefits.

The solution: exercise your penis.

The phrase "use it or lose it" was never more apt than when applied to your penis; absent frequent erections, your penis can actually shrink one to two centimeters. About 70 percent of men who have their prostate removed can expect to lose some penis length. That's why prostate cancer patients, who are often unable to get an erection for six to twenty-four months, are sometimes prescribed penis pumps; that way, they can keep the blood flowing and help prevent permanent shrinkage. Other risk factors for loss of penis length include weight gain, aging (due to lack of use and declining hormones), and genetics.

So how do you exercise your penis? The "love muscle" is actually not a muscle at all, but a shaft of spongy tissue that fills with blood when the time is right. So to keep that tissue in good working order, you need to engage in activities that increase blood flow: namely, regular sex and masturbation.

Not sure if you're still getting those nocturnal erections? Try this simple, urologist-approved test for three nights at home. (Rest assured that I didn't make this up—it's a real test used by urologists, and it has a name, the *nocturnal penile tumescence* (NPT) stamp test. Google it.)

Here's how it works: Get a strip of four to six postage stamps. Wrap the strip around the shaft of your penis and moisten one of the stamps at the end to seal the ring. Once the stamp is dry, carefully place your penis into your shorts or underwear to protect the stamps from falling off.

In the morning, check to see if the stamps have been broken along their perforation. Do this for three nights. During at least one of the three nights you should see the ring of stamps broken. If it isn't, there may be a physical problem, and you should talk to your doctor.

Aside from simply using your penis as much as possible, there are a few medical procedures that can give you more length. All of them, however, come with drawbacks. During penile-enhancement surgery, a doctor releases part of the ligament that attaches your penis to your pelvic bone so more of the penis can move outside the body (about 50 percent of your penis is actually inside your body). It's a serious procedure, so you should look into whether gaining that extra inch or so is worth it.

If girth is more your concern than length, there are some penile-widening procedures as well. A doctor can implant silicone, fat, or tissue grafts into your penis. Another procedure that improves girth is to inject hyaluronic acid into the penis. It is said to be painful but effective.

Maintaining a healthy sex life, though, is the best natural sexercise plan you can follow (along with exercise, diet, and lifestyle modifications). Personally, I don't want anyone cutting or injecting anything into my favorite body part unless there is a serious medical reason for it.

Issue #12: Your PC Needs a Tune-Up

Your PC may need a tune-up. No, not the one you use for Internet porn. The pubococcygeal (PC) muscles in your pelvic floor extend from your anus to your urinary sphincter, serving as a kind of netting across the bones of your pelvis that help hold your internal organs in place. They are also the ones that contract involuntarily during orgasm, and the ones you use to squeeze off the flow of urine when your five-year-old wanders into the bathroom while you're peeing.

Like any other muscle, the PC can lose strength and tone over time—because of nerve damage, excessive sitting, or simply getting older. The good news is, just like any other muscle, you can strengthen the PC with exercise as well—and you don't even need to hit the gym. Kegel exercises—the same ones women do to restore strength in the pelvic floor following childbirth—can improve ED symptoms and help men achieve stronger orgasms, while improving symptoms of incontinence and premature ejaculation as well.

Here's how to do them:

First, find the PC muscles either by imagining stopping the flow of urine or by *actually* stopping urine flow midpee. Take care not to squeeze any other muscles—in your thighs, abdomen, or buttocks—at the same time. With practice, you'll be able to squeeze the PC muscles in your penis separately from those in your anus, which will get you serious PC-muscle control bragging rights.

Once you've mastered the PC squeeze, begin this simple, do-anywhere routine:

- Squeeze the PC muscle.

- Hold for five seconds.

- Release slowly for five seconds.

- Repeat twelve to fifteen times, up to three times a day.

Some men get crazy with Kegels, placing a light towel over their erect penises for resistance and lifting the towel with each rep. Sounds extreme to me, but if you're that excited about building PC muscles that could outsqueeze a boa constrictor, knock yourself out.

Issue #13: You Need a Pill to Get Going

If all else fails, the famous little blue pill Viagra—and its main competitors, Cialis and Levitra—can restore blood flow to the penis. But before you go this route, give natural remedies a serious try first. This isn't just my innate distrust of blockbuster medications talking (though that's something I'm definitely guilty of). I also recommend the other natural measures because taking any of the ones mentioned earlier will improve the state of your health generally—and better erections will be a positive side effect. In the medical community, "ED" stands not just for erectile dysfunction but for "early death": a signpost for a more serious, potentially terminal, issue in your future. Don't accept it as an inevitable part of getting older; instead, use it as motivation to make changes elsewhere in your life that will solve the current problem and avoid serious problems down the line.

Like falling asleep—or, indeed, falling in love—an erection isn't something you can *make* happen; more commonly, it just happens when the circumstances are right. So there are times when you may fall into an erection rut, psyching yourself out right when you should be getting busy. It's a little like getting the yips in golf: you remember that you had problems last time, start to worry that you might have them again, and pretty soon, the worry itself becomes the issue. If that's the case for you, pills can be a good way to get yourself back on the sex track. Once your confidence is back, drop the blue pills . . . and see if the blue steel returns.

HOW ED PILLS WORK

I've already gone over the basic process of how erections occur. Essentially it's a multi-phase chemical domino effect:

- You catch sight of something that turns you on—and you get aroused.

- Your brain sends neural signals to the *corpora cavernosa*, two spongy tubes that run along the length of the penis . . .

- which in turn produce *nitric oxide* . . .

- which in turn stimulates an enzyme called *guanylate cyclase* . . .

- which transforms a chemical called GTP into another chemical called cGMP. cGMP is a major player here because it relaxes the smooth muscle in the arteries, allowing blood flow in the penis to increase. Meanwhile, the veins that carry blood out of the penis constrict, trapping blood in the corpora cavernosa.

- Bango—you're all charged up and ready for action.

Also involved in this neurochemical assembly line is another chemical called PDE5, which converts cGMP back into GTP. When that happens, it's wet noodle time, because you can't cowboy up without plenty of cGMP.

ED medications like Viagra are PDE5-*inhibitors*: they inhibit the stuff that inhibits an erection. Once it's attached to the PDE5 in the penis, the chemical can't break down the cGMP anymore, and you're off to the races again.

None of this is possible, however, without that initial sexual stimulus from the brain. Pound as many blue pills as you like, but your penis won't jump into action unless your brain is on board and sexually aroused. As with so many other things, an erection is in the head—and in the heart.

Issue #14: You've Got the Blues

Depression, which can also wreak havoc on your autonomic nervous system, can be an insidious erection-killer, winding you up, or equally, quashing you down, so much so that you can't rise appropriately to the occasion. Unfortunately, antidepressants, which can be effective in staving off the anxiety and listlessness associated with depression, can themselves cause erectile problems, leading to a Catch-22: Go off the meds so you can get your performance back, and risk a depressive crash? Or stay on them to keep your mood elevated, and accept the performance issues as an unfortunate price to pay?

I can't speak from personal experience on this, and I realize that for some people, the pills can be lifesaving. But there is compelling evidence that, for many depressed people, regular exercise may be the best medication of all. One 2011 study found that "exercise and physical activity have beneficial effects on depression symptoms that are comparable to those of antidepressant treatments." Other studies have found that in the long term, exercise may be even more effective at preventing relapses in depression. Perhaps this is because it's an active, rather than a passive, intervention that you yourself control, and feeling out of control—and at the mercy of mysterious chemicals coursing through your body—is one of the major reasons people get depressed in the first place. By exercising to alleviate depression, you're taking charge, seizing control in a situation in which you can feel very disempowered. The additional benefit to exercising your way out of a depressive state, of course, is that rather than causing ED, exercise helps get rid of it.

Needless to say, make sure you talk it over with your physician if you are considering going off any type of medication.

Issue #15: You're Under Surveillance

Back when I was forty, as a result of an elevated PSA level in a blood test, a urologist put me on an "active surveillance" program that required me to be subjected to biannual prostate biopsies. Little did I know that this nasty little procedure—designed to detect prostate cancer—ironically carried the risk of causing erectile dysfunction, sometimes for the long term.

This, by the way, is also true of Proscar, Flomax, and a number of other drugs designed to alleviate an enlarged prostate. Propecia, a similar drug, is also used as a treatment for baldness—so take care when picking your poison.

Other possible side effects of these biopsies include ejaculatory problems and infertility—a particularly cruel irony since these are procedures and drugs that purport to help keep your plumbing in good working order (and your hair looking great).

There are various ways to perform a biopsy, and some urologists are more aggressive than others with the number of needles they insert to take tissue samples. Studies indicate that the more frequent and more intense the biopsies, and the more insertions the doctor performs, the more likely the biopsies are to cause ED.

After enduring two biopsies over six months, I ultimately went against my urologist's recommendations and opted for naturopathic remedies and immaculate self-care rather than more potential prostate trauma and potential erectile problems. And I'm incredibly glad I did. Working with a more progressive doctor, I brought my PSA levels down into the normal range and no longer worry as much about prostate cancer.

I would point out, though, that a prostate biopsy is the only current method available to determine the degree and stage of prostate cancer in men—so for some of us, it's unavoidable. I personally decided that the risks associated with the procedure designed to identify the disease were almost as bad as the disease itself—and found a smart, well-informed doctor who agreed with my course of action and helped me with an alternate plan. If that option is available to you, I'd advise you to take a similar path.

The good news? Twelve weeks postprocedure, the vast majority of men who undergo even the most invasive biopsies usually regain their lost sexual functioning. A single biopsy is unlikely to cause long-term problems. If you need them regularly, however, find a urologist who will listen to your very legitimate concerns. And ask for an MRI-guided biopsy, a new imaging procedure that allows more targeted biopsies and better identification of potential tumors.

And if you are on Flomax or Proscar for an enlarged prostate, remember that some of the sexual side effects may persist for up to two years after you stop taking the drugs—so work with your urologist to get off them as soon as you are able.

Issue #16: You Spend Too Much Time in the Saddle

Nearly 2,500 years ago, Hippocrates noted of the Scythians, a tribe known for their horsemanship, "The constant jolting on their horses unfits them for intercourse." It's probably still true of equestrians, but today it's even more true of avid cyclists. Cycling three hours a week or more causes a steep increase in the rates of ED, one German study found. The reason should be obvious: when you ride a bike, much of your weight rests on your perineum, the soft, fleshy channel between your scrotum and anus through which the main artery that supplies blood to your penis runs. Sitting on this vulnerable spot long enough causes blood flow to your genitals to drop up to 80 percent. It also puts you at increased risk for prostatitis, an inflammation of the prostate, and another condition called "chronic pelvic pain syndrome"—which is exactly as nasty as it sounds.

Most erectile issues seem to accrue with three or more hours of riding per week. So if you're a casual bike commuter, or if you like to jump on your bike with your kids now and again, you're probably not at much risk. It's guys who do two hours a day and four on Sundays who are most at risk.

SAY YES TO NO

Nitric oxide (NO) is a molecule in the body that has a huge impact on sexual performance. It's produced in the endothelial lining, the microscopically thin inner layer of cells that wallpaper the inside of all your blood vessels, from the biggest arteries to the tiniest capillaries. NO circulates as a gas—meaning that when it hits, it hits hard and fast, and you feel its effects everywhere.

The triggers for NO are some of our favorite feel-good activities like working out and having sex. Pick up a barbell, or grab your partner for a sexual romp, and you get flushed because NO is forcing your blood vessels to enlarge, increasing circulation in the muscles, face, and, yes, the penis. At the same time, NO regulates the levels of numerous neurotransmitters in the body, lowering inflammation, improving the health of the heart, and balancing adrenal levels. NO, then, is a key ingredient not only in facilitating sex itself but also in enhancing the body's positive, health-boosting response to sex as well.

As is the case with many other hormones, NO production tends to drop off as we get older. By the age of forty, most of us produce only about half the NO we produced in our twenties. But a number of foods can enhance NO production, and thus circulatory health and potency as well: arugula, beets, celery, chervil, lettuce, spinach, and watercress all contain more than 250 milligrams of nitrates per 100 grams (3.5 ounces). Chinese cabbage, endive, celeriac, fennel, leeks, and parsley all contain 100 milligrams per 100 grams. Blackberries, bilberries, and elderberries can provide erection protection too: they contain high levels of antioxidants called *anthocyanins*, which fight free radicals that can interfere with NO production.

Other good choices:

- all leafy green vegetables
- dark chocolate
- watermelon
- walnuts
- pomegranate
- brown rice
- oranges
- cranberries

- black tea
- cayenne pepper
- honey
- pistachios
- salmon
- garlic
- onions

Many of these foods are feel-good options that also boost testosterone and heart health. So keep them on the menu, and it won't be just your sex life that's flying high, but your head-to-toe vitality as well.

If this is you, and you're not willing to curb your time in the saddle, at least change positions often when you ride so that you don't put constant pressure on the same delicate tissue. Also, invest in a seat with no nose, which allows you to put weight on your sitting bones and eliminates pressure on the perineum (grooved bicycle seats, which were designed to address the problem, may actually make it worse, as the arteries that supply blood to the penis don't run straight down the center of the perineum). Noseless seats are pretty novel (some of them look like two Mickey Mouse ears), but I'm going to guess they'll become the norm in the next few years. Protect your plumbing by getting on the forefront of this trend.

Finally: if you absolutely, positively must ride a bike for hours and hours every week, at least take a break in the seventy-two hours before a PSA test. Cycling can spike PSA levels and give a false indication of possible prostate cancer—not a scare you want to have to weather.

PROSTATE HEALTH: PROTECTING YOUR THIRD NUT

If you've reached Your New Prime and haven't had a compelling reason to learn all about your prostate, consider yourself lucky. At present, benign prostatic hyperplasia—the enlargement of the prostate—is roughly as common as heart disease or diabetes. Fifty percent of men over fifty and 60 percent of men over sixty get up more than twice a night to pee due to an enlarged prostate. And one in six men will develop prostate cancer. The lack of sleep—and anxiety—caused by these issues can spiral into chronic stress, weight gain, lack of exercise, low testosterone, and poor appetite regulation—all those things that guys over forty are trying so hard to avoid. So for men, prostate issues can be a vicious cycle.

As with a head gasket or a carburetor, you generally know about the prostate only when there's something wrong with it. So here's a little primer: The prostate is a walnut-size gland located below the bladder. It wraps around the urethra, the tube that runs through the penis and eventually serves as the exit point for semen (and urine). The prostate, then, is right in the middle of the action.

Fundamentally, the prostate's job is to be a caretaker for your sperm. It produces alkaline seminal fluid, which protects the sperm during its journey through the acidity of the vaginal canal. The gland also helps filter various toxins out of seminal fluid and protects against urinary tract infections.

The prostate also produces prostate-specific antigen (PSA), which helps keep sperm in liquid form; it also plays a role in achieving an erection, controlling urine flow, and intensifying sexual pleasure.

Not bad for one little gland.

Needless to say, then, keeping this third nut up and running well is pretty important to the New Primer's quality of life. Some of the potential issues that can affect the prostate include:

- Growing larger than normal. When this happens, the prostate can push against the bladder from below, causing an incomplete flushing out of the bladder during urination. This in turn can cause urinary tract infections and frequent, and urgent, trips to the bathroom.

- Squeezing the urethra. Step lightly on a garden hose and you'll slow the flow of water from the nozzle; step more heavily and you can stop the flow entirely. Either scenario is possible when the prostate compresses the urethra.

- Developing cancer. Prostate cancer affects one out of six men. Though relatively slow-growing, prostate cancer can spread to other tissues in the body—the bladder, liver, brain, and elsewhere—where it can cause more damage.

Most of the urinary symptoms that keep us up at night develop as a result of *benign prostatic hyperplasia (BPH)*, a noncancerous overproliferation of prostate cells, or *prostatitis*, an inflammation or infection in the prostate, which affects nearly half of all men at some point. Prostate cancer symptoms can be similar to BPH or prostatitis, but most men find out they have prostate cancer only as the result of a routine examination—which is why it is important to get screened regularly once you hit forty.

All three conditions share similar symptoms, and most of them have to do with how often—and how urgently—you take trips to the men's room. A few of the issues include:

- having to wait for the urinary stream to begin

- urinary flow starting and stopping

- weak urinary stream

- dribbling urine

- frequent need to urinate

- incomplete urination (or inability to completely empty the bladder)

- urgent need to urinate

- urinary tract infections

- urinary incontinence (leakage)

- inability to urinate (an emergency situation)

Prostatitis may also cause pain during ejaculation and pain in the genital or pelvic area generally; prostate cancer, depending on how advanced it is, may cause numerous other issues, including weight loss, anemia, bloody semen or urine, lower back or abdominal pain, and fatigue.

Your New Prime lifestyle is your first line of defense in improving the symptoms of poor prostate health and in preventing problems altogether. Key among the behaviors that will keep your prostate healthy are the following:

Reduce Sedentary Time

Things like exercise, taking breaks from sitting at work, and stand-up workstations are examples of concrete steps you can take to improve your prostate health through reducing sedentary time. In a 2014 study of nearly six hundred men, those who sat between 4.5 and 7 hours a day (those with lower levels of sedentary time) had "a significantly lower risk of BPH than those with a higher sedentary time (7 hours or more)."

Consume Foods with Anti-inflammatory Properties

Eating anti-inflammatory foods, such as fruits, cruciferous veggies, vegetable proteins, and other foods discussed in chapter 3, can reduce both inflammation and the risk of developing BPH. Some of my personal favorites—like kale, green tea, tomatoes, olive oil, dark chocolate, and berries—are also *antiangiogenic*: they fight cancer by preventing the growth of the blood vessels that feed tumors.

Work Out

A recent study found that men who walked—or performed equally mild forms of exercise—just one to three hours a week had an 86 percent lower chance of contracting a deadly form of prostate cancer than men who were entirely sedentary. That means that even a small amount of mild exercise can help reduce your risk. A different study showed that three to six hours a week of exercise resulted in a significant reduction in the risk of all types of prostate cancer. Studies have also indicated that exercise—a global anti-inflammatory—can significantly reduce the symptoms of prostatitis and BPH as well.

Live Clean

Unsurprisingly, alcohol, smoking, and poor sleep habits can adversely affect your prostate—just as they affect every other system in the body. Conversely, homeopathic treatments like massage, progressive relaxation, acupuncture, stress management, and other self-care methods can boost prostate health. Smart self-care is smart prostate care.

Get It On

The *Journal of the American Medical Association* reported recently that men who had more than twenty ejaculations per month (through sexual activity, masturbation, or wet dreams—remember those?) were 33 percent less likely to develop prostate cancer than those who had fewer ejaculations. A 2009 study corroborated the finding, concluding that ten or more sexual encounters per month bestowed a small amount of protection against the disease. Just be sure to avoid sex in the seventy-two hours before a PSA test, as doing the wild thing can artificially elevate your levels.

Supplement Your Life

As you know, I'm a supplement guy—always researching and experimenting with the best and latest supplements for all manner of ailments. As with many other conditions, there are lots of supplements out there purporting to improve prostate health, and a few that actually seem to work.

The duds include *lycopene*, which is popular but does nothing for the prostate. *Saw palmetto* can confer other benefits but is no better than a placebo, based on the largest and most recent study. Better choices are supplements with proven anti-inflammatory properties. Some of my favorites that are supported by clinical studies include:

- bee pollen/cernilton
- quercetin
- beta sitosterol
- turmeric/curcumin
- vitamin D3
- Pygeum africanum
- stinging nettle
- green tea extract
- cranberry
- diindolylmethane (DIM)
- cayenne/capsaicin

NINE TESTS EVERY MAN OVER FORTY SHOULD TAKE

Most men avoid going to the doctor unless they're dragged there by a family member when things get serious. I have spoken to dozens of men with prostate or colon cancer who avoided going to the doctor—sometimes for decades—out of fear of some of these tests.

But getting tested on a regular basis is essential—especially as you age. The following are tests that every man over forty should have done, as they may help you detect silent killers such as high blood pressure, or catch or even reverse other diseases while they are still in their early, treatable stages. Get these done and don't mess around.

PSA

The PSA test measures the level of prostate-specific antigen, an indicator of prostate health in your blood. A rising or high PSA may indicate prostate cancer, or it could point to another prostate condition that may need medical attention, or it may itself lead to cancer. Despite some controversy surrounding this test, it is still an important test for all men to consider as an early warning of reduced prostate health. I found out I had an abnormally high PSA about a decade ago after a PSA blood test. Since then, I have massively changed certain aspects of my diet and lifestyle to prevent any potential progression to prostate cancer—and today my PSA level is below normal for my age.

DRE

The digital rectal exam (DRE) is a simple procedure for the early detection and diagnosis of prostate cancer and other abnormalities of the prostate gland. The doctor inserts a lubricated gloved finger in the rectum to feel the prostate gland for lumps or enlargement. As such, it's the test guys fear the most. But man up and have it done, because it could save your life.

TESTOSTERONE

Low T can cause several changes such as erectile dysfunction, fatigue, weight gain, loss of muscle, loss of body hair, sleep problems, trouble concentrating, bone loss, and personality changes. Your doctor can check your testosterone through a blood or saliva test. Before you jump on the T therapy wagon, though, I urge you to read the recommendations in chapters 1 and 2.

BONE DENSITY

Osteoporosis may be more common in women, but men get it too. Experts recommend that men over fifty who are in high-risk groups (low T, family history, sedentary lifestyle, smokers, etc.) get tested, and men of normal risk get tested at sixty. A bone density scan (DEXA) can measure how strong your bones are and help you determine the risk of a fracture.

CHOLESTEROL

There are different kinds of cholesterol circulating in your blood. When you get tested you should receive the following measures:

- total cholesterol;
- low-density lipoprotein (LDL) or your "bad" cholesterol;
- high-density lipoprotein (HDL) or your "good" cholesterol; and your
- triglycerides, which are another form of fat in the blood.

High cholesterol is one of the risk factors for heart disease. Most men can have their cholesterol tested as part of a routine blood test.

BLOOD PRESSURE

Blood pressure is a silent killer. You should have it checked every two years unless your doctor recommends that you get it checked more regularly. There are no symptoms of high blood pressure, but it can harm your heart, lungs, brain, kidneys, and blood vessels.

BLOOD SUGAR

A blood sugar test measures the amount of glucose in your blood. The test is an important screening for diabetes or prediabetes and insulin resistance. Untreated diabetes will continue to get worse and cause problems with eyes, feet, heart, skin, mental health, nerves, kidneys, and more. Insulin resistance causes weight gain, high blood pressure, high cholesterol, bloating, and high blood sugar. When untreated, it can lead to diabetes. Although I'm not diabetic, I regularly take my blood sugar with a home blood sugar monitor so I can keep an eye on my glucose levels.

COLORECTAL CANCER SCREENING

Doctors recommend that people ages fifty to seventy-five get screened for colon cancer with any of three following tests: the sigmoidoscopy, colonoscopy, and the fecal occult blood test.

The US Multi-Society Task Force on Colorectal Cancer has ranked the screening methods. They say that tests like fecal occult blood screens can detect early stage cancers, but the colonoscopy is considered the best test for prevention.

I have a history of colon cancer, as my mom died from the disease in her early seventies, so I started getting checked every three to four years starting when I was forty. So far, so good—and it's worth the regular screening to know for sure.

HIV TEST

You may be surprised to see HIV on the list, but about 15 percent of new infections each year are among people over age fifty, and people over fifty represent almost one-fourth of the HIV/AIDS cases in the United States. With birth control no longer a concern, many people over age fifty are having unprotected sex. Doctors don't usually ask their older patients about sex, and educational programs that teach prevention neglect the patients in this age group—but HIV is certainly still a concern no matter how old you are.

These nine tests can help you stay healthy and improve your longevity. By giving you a warning that you have a condition that puts you at risk of a more serious disease, they can allow you to make changes in your diet, exercise, and other habits to reduce your risks. Because some of these conditions have no symptoms, you may have no idea that you have a problem if you do not get tested. It is easier and less expensive to prevent disease than to try to treat it after years of damage have set in.

Sexual health, like sex itself, is a whole-self endeavor—part emotional, part physical, part intellectual, part biological, part creative. Some even find it a spiritual experience. Unlike, say, your exercise routine, it's also not just about you—it's about a mysterious coming together, both literally and figuratively, of you and another person.

As such, cultivating a gratifying sex life is rather more complex than any five-point action plan on getting more and giving more that some "sexperts" promise. That's why this chapter contains so many distinct pieces of advice. And that's also what makes sex so endlessly fascinating: try as we might, we can't "hack" sex. It will always remain somewhat elusive and unknowable, just like our partners themselves. And I consider that something to celebrate.

YOUR THIRTY-DAY ACTION PLAN FOR BETTER SEXUAL HEALTH

Sexual health—and an exciting, satisfying sex life—depends on a host of factors that are both psychological and physiological. To start getting yours up to snuff, put these body-mind techniques to work over the next thirty days:

Psychological

1. **Focus on your partner's needs** both in and out of the bedroom.

2. **Be amenable to having sex** with your partner, even if you aren't into it first.

3. **Instigate a forty-eight-hour rule:** At least every forty-eight hours, one of you must initiate sex with the other. Alternate who initiates.

4. **Pay attention to the little things** and appreciate your partner for what she does for you.

5. **Trust the comings and goings of sexual desire** over the years of a long-term relationship.

6. **Give your partner space**, and take it for yourself when you need it.

7. **Ask—tactfully—for what you need** in the bedroom.

8. **Appreciate one another's bodies** in nonsexual ways, especially by exercising together.

9. If you exercise compulsively, **also spend some time doing yoga**, particularly with your partner.

10. **Monitor (and moderate, if necessary) your use of porn.**

Physical

11. **Clean up your diet** (see chapter 3).

12. **Work on losing weight** if necessary (see chapter 4).

13. **Consider using potency-enhancing supplements** like EveryDay Male.

14. **Exercise**, focusing on movements that elevate your heart rate.

15. **Don't smoke.**

16. **Spend more time on de-stressing activities.**

17. **Consider acupuncture.**

18. **Ease up on alcohol.**

19. **Detox your home.**

20. **Perform Kegel exercises** to develop the muscles of your pelvic floor.

21. Experiment with exercise as a natural antidepressant.

22. If you're under watchful surveillance for prostate cancer, **discuss lifestyle interventions, and less invasive monitoring options, with your doctor.** If frequent and intense biopsies are presented as your only option, consider changing physicians.

23. Cycle no more than three hours per week.

24. Consume NO-enhancing foods.

CHAPTER 6

The Head Trip

Optimizing Brainpower

There is nothing either good or bad, but thinking makes it so.

—WILLIAM SHAKESPEARE, *HAMLET*

ALL IN YOUR HEAD

"It's all in your head."

We hear this phrase all the time: from well-meaning physicians, from our kids, from our spouses and friends. Worried that the boss doesn't like you? *That's all in your head.* Afraid you're getting sick? *Your mind is playing tricks on you.* Worried you're slowing down, losing your edge, falling out of touch with your family? *You're imagining things.*

Usually, when people tell us this, they're trying to reassure us that, whatever our *perception* of a situation, in *reality*, everything is fine. Quit worrying. You're making it all up.

The problem, as Shakespeare so concisely pointed out, is that perception is everything. What's in your head makes its way into the decisions you make, big, small, and everywhere in between. I'm writing these words just a few weeks after the actor Robin Williams—a vigorous guy who had more fame, wealth, and adulation than most men could hope for—committed suicide. From the outside, Williams's life appeared abundant, laudable, and inspiring. We now know that for Williams, tragically, his life was another story. And we hear of similar incidents all the time.

On the flip side, I have known people who have suffered horrible traumas—cancer, prison, destitute poverty, concentration camps—who have emerged remarkably positive and effective, who rarely if ever seem sullen or depressed. I imagine you have as well. An older woman I know spent over a year in a hayloft hiding from the Nazis in France. Much of her family was killed in the war. Later, as a young teen, she was in a coma for a full year. And yet Michelle is engaged, positive, and spilling over with vitality and good cheer. Perception *is* reality, as much so for irrepressibly positive people as for the ones who go off the deep end when they seem to have it all.

But it isn't just mood and outlook that are affected by our thinking. Our bodies are profoundly affected by it as well. The placebo effect, which posits that a person's belief in a treatment, medicine, practitioner, or practice greatly influences its efficacy, has been studied for centuries, and it has been shown to be remarkably and consistently potent. One compelling example among many: A 2002 study of people with osteoarthritis found that "sham" surgery—in which patients received an incision and a faked procedure—was no less effective than arthroscopic surgery, or another accepted treatment called lavage, for curing knee pain. Though it's common knowledge that fake pills can influence health, this study made it clear that fake surgery can too. In essence, the patients *made up their minds that they were cured*—and that decision, on its own, cured them. As the saying goes, the mind works in mysterious ways, including fixing a problem in the body that most physicians would consider largely mechanical.

Here's another example of the power of thinking, this one perhaps even stranger: Back in 1981, eight men, all in their seventies and in various stages of declining health, spent five days in an elaborately formulated "time warp" monastery. The living space was designed to invoke the year 1959, when the men were in their fifties. While there, the men were instructed to behave as if it were 1959 again. They discussed sports heroes, movies, and world events of that era. Mirrors were forbidden, as were modern clothes and all photos of themselves after 1959.

Shockingly, after just five days, the men were more dexterous, mentally sharper and suppler, and they had better posture. They appeared younger. Their eyesight improved. And they outperformed a similar group of men who had taken a five-day rest cure without the time warp intervention.

It's a small study, but a well-conducted one, and the implications are huge: the physical effects of aging, while perhaps not *all* in your head, are clearly subject to suggestion, behavior, and outlook. In this case, if you believe yourself to be young, vigorous, engaged, and relevant, and behave as if you are—you will be.

My friend Kelly Slater, a legendary competitive surfer who at forty-three still regularly bests far younger men, says of his unusual longevity in the sport, "I'm healthy, and I'm competing with guys who are literally half my age or less. I don't personally tie anything to that. I don't care what my age is. These are my peers and I'm surfing against them. If they have a problem that I'm older, then go ahead and beat me." He doesn't consider his age a limitation. And so, for all intents and purposes, it isn't.

The upshot: It's quite possible that the way we see the world, and our place in it, may be at least as important to our health and well-being as whatever may actually be going on in our bodies and in our lives. Study after study, as well as our day-to-day personal experience, is proving that all the time.

True as that may be, however, it begs an important question: *How do I improve my outlook?* And that's what this chapter is about: giving you mental techniques that will make you sharper, more positive, happier, and more effective (and thereby, as the accounts earlier in this chapter indicate, physically healthier). All well and good, I hear you say. I would be happier. I would improve my outlook. But first I need a bigger house. More holidays in Tahiti. A bigger retirement account. A Ferrari. We often believe we need something *external* to help us achieve these benefits, and for many of us, that external thing is the green stuff you keep in a bank.

Far be it from me to tell you not to go after and enjoy material comforts: I like a nice car, a nice house, and lots of money as much as the next guy. But there is plenty of evidence to suggest that seeking external things to supply us with happiness is a fool's errand.

Given all the time we put into worrying about whether we have enough of it and how we might get more of it, wealth, as it turns out, affects happiness much less than we think it does. Consider: In a 2013 study, people who made just over $13,000 a year rated their happiness, on a scale of one to ten, at just under a seven. But people who made $120,000 a year rated their happiness *only one point higher*, at just under an eight. To state the obvious, going from $13K to $120K a year is an enormous reversal of fortune—a near-tenfold increase in wealth. A person who managed such a jump in income would be rocketing from one step above abject poverty to the top 12 percent of wage earners worldwide. He may pay off a home, buy a car or two, and eat out at dinner more. But such a person *wouldn't* get a substantial bump in happiness. And the bump he would get would be far out of proportion to the level of happiness most of us think such a huge increase in personal wealth would impart.

So happiness comes from somewhere else, and we've got to start looking for it outside of our bottom line if we ever want to achieve it.

The positive side of "it's all in your head" is that, to a large extent, we have absolute power over what we think. Indeed, it may be the one area in which we do have near-total control—if we choose to exert that influence rather than letting old habits, patterns, and foregone conclusions rule us from the inside out. If happiness and contentment are largely a matter of what goes on in our gray matter, then making conscious choices about what goes on in there—no less than the conscious choices we make about how we eat and exercise—may be the most important step we can take in our New Prime to ensure lasting health and contentment.

This chapter will cover the best practices on how to make that happen for yourself. Because happiness is inextricably connected to your external circumstances and your physical vitality, the techniques (if we can call them that) are both internal and external: some address the way you think about your life, and some address the way you do your life. As we'll see, these approaches are not altogether separate.

THE MENTAL HEALTH AUDIT

1. Do you often spend a half hour or more per night—before falling asleep or in the middle of the night—worrying about your career, finances, relationships, or other crises you don't feel you can control?

2. Do you feel out of control of your life?

3. Do you spend less than 30 percent of your time doing activities you genuinely enjoy (whether they are related to work, hobbies, or family activities)?

4. Do you have one or more big life projects (a business you'd like to start, a big trip you'd like to take) you've always wanted to start, but haven't?

5. Do you worry that stress is affecting your health?

6. Do you spend less than ten minutes a day in some form of meditative practice?

7. Do you spend less than ten minutes a day on activities specifically to reduce stress in your life?

8. Do you spend more than 30 percent of your time engaged in activities you dislike?

9. Do you believe that more money would fundamentally alter your happiness level?

10. Do you sleep less than six hours—or more than eight hours—most nights?

11. Is your memory less dependable than it used to be?

12. Are you unclear about what positive steps you could be taking toward your next life goal?

13. Do you spend a lot of your working day with two or more active "screens" open?

14. Are you frequently confused about how to order and prioritize your to-do list?

15. Do you believe that smart nutrition and exercise practices can compensate for poor sleep habits, lack of social connection, and a high-stress lifestyle?

16. Do you have three or more close friends outside of your family to whom you have—or could have—turned in an emergency? Have these same people turned to you under similar circumstances?

17. Do you think about the life you want to be leading in five, ten, or twenty years?

"Yes" answers on questions 1–15 suggest that your mental health practices could use a brushup, and "no" answers on questions 16 and 17 indicates the same. And mental health is important regardless of how scrupulously you take care of your body.

BRAINPOWER TIP #1: REFRAME THE MIDLIFE CRISIS

Around age forty-five or fifty, many men experience a midlife crisis.

I probably don't need to define this delightful little phenomenon for you, but just to make sure we're talking about the same thing, a midlife crisis is a period, usually falling during our fifth or sixth decade, of feeling rudderless, at sea, and unfocused. Many men question decisions that they made in the past. *Why did I ever decide to pursue medicine?* thinks the overworked, forty-two-year-old doctor, itching to try another vocation. *Why did I marry so young?* thinks the stressed-out forty-six-year-old husband, wondering about all the women he missed out on dating. *Why did I spend so much money when I was younger?* thinks the fifty-four-year-old banker, worrying about retirement.

As I've mentioned, Your New Prime can be a big, fat reckoning period, and few of us will be 100 percent comfortable with the final bill. We're constantly wrapped up in "grass is greener" thinking. You look over your life and the choices you've made and you wonder "What was I thinking?" or "What could or should I have done—and why didn't I?"

It's probably useful to remember, however, that you weren't the one doing the thinking at the time. At twenty-five, perhaps the career you chose, or the woman you married, or the city you settled in, were, in fact, perfect for you. But as much as you may be loath to admit it, *you're not twenty-five anymore.* You have learned lessons. You have different priorities. What once was challenging for you may now be relatively dull. Part of you—an important, wise part of you—may very well have moved on. The midlife "crisis," then, is the point at which the choices you've made feel intractable—and the distance between the life you've built for yourself and the life you now want can feel insurmountable. Simultaneously, there's the very real (and very accurate!) feeling that someday, in what's starting to feel like the not-too-distant future, you're going to have to pick up your bat and ball and go home.

And that, my friend, is the midlife crisis: a profound feeling that something needs to change in a major way—and that time is running out.

Playing the sociological commentator for a moment, I'll offer that I think we're up against some pretty serious and misguided cultural forces in midlife. In our youth-obsessed culture, we are expected, it seems, to drift slowly into resigned irrelevance as middle age sets in. But this idea that we're supposed to go out to pasture in middle age runs completely contrary to the natural order of things. In indigenous societies, for example, age, and the experience and wisdom that come with it, are held in reverence. Elders, with their long, personal memory of the comings and goings of the forces that affect and shape our lives, are always the leaders in those communities—and the younger people the willing followers. A forty-three-year-old friend of mine recently went to a Native American reservation in Colorado to shoot a documentary film. The elders of the village were incredulous—and amused to the point of laughter—that someone so young would be in charge of such an important project.

So I'll repeat here my belief that what we call the midlife crisis is actually a very good thing. It's you wanting to step into your rightful role as a revered and respected tribal elder. It's you raging against the dying of the light. It's you wanting to grow and change and evolve with the passion and dynamism of your younger self. It's you wanting to stay physically and mentally vibrant and energetic. It's you wanting to hazard yourself boldly in the world, resisting, with every fiber of your being, this culture's desire to shove you aside and make room for younger generations.

Rather than flailing around, looking for novelty wherever you can find it (career, finances, relationships), you should embrace midlife as an excellent opportunity—perhaps the best one you'll ever have—to look *inward*, to reestablish your connection with what you do well and to decide how you want to practice and share those strengths with the world. Yes, time is tighter than it was when you were twenty. But you also know yourself better. You know your passion, ambitions, desires, and abilities better than you ever did, and you now have a wealth of experiences that you can bring to bear on your next steps, whatever they may be.

Instead of letting midlife cause you to panic and collapse, seize this period as the chance to get laser-focused on what you want to do, and who you want to be, for the second half (or two-thirds!) of your life.

WHY THE OVER-FORTY CROWD STILL MATTERS (A LOT)

In Tom Robbins's great book *Jitterbug Perfume*, there's a reference to the old days when the chief of the tribe was executed at the first sign of a gray hair on his head.

Sometimes being over forty can feel like that (hell, twenty-five feels old in Silicon Valley). But the actual statistics suggest otherwise. The truth is that we're an enormous, vital, and financially secure (read: powerful and influential) group. Consider the following facts about the United States:

- There are ninety million boomers and seniors in the United States alone.
- An American turns fifty every seven seconds—more than 12,500 each day.
- As of 2015, people aged fifty to seventy-five will represent 40 percent of US adult consumers.
- The fifty-plus audience is the largest demographic in history—and will be for the next fifty years.

- The US Census projects a 75 percent increase in the population aged sixty-five and older by 2030.

- In 2011, the first boomers turned sixty-five.

- The last of the boomer population will turn 65 in 2030.

- People over fifty have over $2.4 trillion in annual income.

- The fifty-plus segment is the most affluent consumer group today.

- Over the past decade, the highest rate of new business creation has been posted by those aged fifty-five to sixty-four.

- In 2012, almost a quarter of new businesses were started by entrepreneurs fifty-five and older—a 14 percent spike since 1996.

- Adults aged fifty-plus spend an average of $7 billion online annually.

- More than 50 percent of discretionary spending power belongs to boomers.

- The fifty-plus age group owns over 80 percent of the money in savings accounts.

- Discretionary income goes up $5,000 when kids leave the house.

- Baby boomers are 26 percent of the population but 40 percent of the economy.

I look at these numbers and I see a group that has been hugely successful and continues to remain hugely relevant. I see a group that's the primary driving force of the economy, one whose ideas still have the power to change the course of society. We have experience, we have capital, and we have vision.

Ray Kroc was fifty-two when he went into business with the McDonald brothers to start a little restaurant chain called McDonald's. Harlan Sanders started franchising Kentucky Fried Chicken at age sixty-five. And Momofuko Ando, the inventor of ramen noodles, started selling precooked instant noodles at age forty-eight.

If I wanted to start another business, I'd market it to this group—and if I wanted to go into business with someone, I'd choose someone in this group. We know our passions, and we know our strengths and weaknesses.

My point: If you're over forty—even well over forty—it's not too late to change, to start a business, or to pursue audacious goals. You still have an important voice. Your ideas, your passions, and your points of view matter. Don't let fear of an ageist society silence you, or keep you from going after what you want.

BRAINPOWER TIP #2: MAP YOUR COURSE FORWARD

So how do you reset your course, focus on a new goal, and change a life that's starting to seem irreversibly set in its ways?

It's simple: one step at a time.

I believe the typical midlife spinout (affair, sports car, job performance spiral, addiction, trouble with kids and marriage) happens when we allow our desire for change to build to a critical and dangerous head. Rather than recognizing at age forty that we want to pivot our lives toward some new endeavor and taking active steps in that direction, we stew about what we're *not* doing, and the life we're *not* living, for many years. Finally we explode, thinking that everything needs to change at once. And the sad result is often a broken marriage, family chaos, and misguided career upheaval.

I'm not saying that drastic and dramatic action is never warranted. Some men have been so miserable for so long that it's the only choice they have, and, after a stormy period, they do find happiness with a different life partner, a different career, or both.

Instead of taking the nuclear option, however, I submit that what's really needed for most of us who are experiencing midlife restlessness is to take honest stock. What's the thing you really want to spend more time doing? Playing music? Designing software? Starting your own business? Skiing, surfing, writing novels, climbing snow-capped peaks, sailing? And then decide—strategically and practically—how you can work those activities into your life.

Figuring out the next big step in your personal evolution can in fact be the toughest step of all.

I hear the protests: *But I don't have time/money/resources/support. If I'm going to write a novel, I need a cabin in the woods, a six-month leave from work, half a million dollars, and paid-up child care the whole time. It's impossible, and I'll never do it.*

It isn't impossible, and whether you do it or not is entirely up to you—not your external circumstances. Chances are you need a lot less than you think you need. I know a man who wrote an award-winning play while living in a studio apartment in Manhattan with two roommates and working as a short-order cook. There was so much distracting city noise from below that he had to wear two pairs of earmuffs as he wrote (he couldn't even afford fancy noise-canceling headphones). But he made it happen. The Life Is Good apparel company, now worth over $100 million, was started by two brothers in Boston with $78 in the bank. Starbucks was started by a couple of teachers and a writer. Mattel, Facebook, Subway, Hewlett-Packard, and Apple Computers were all started by people of average means fooling around with ways to make innovative products in their spare time.

So you don't need all the time and resources in the world to get started on a life-changing project. In fact, too much space, money, and time at the beginning of a big project can overwhelm and smother the spark that gave it life to begin with. There's a good chance that, given that cabin in the woods and all the money he needed, our hypothetical wannabe novelist would fritter away all that time and have nothing to show for it after six months.

Rather than tossing a hand grenade into the life you've built, start with one simple, real step toward a change you want to see, and make it a regular practice. A half hour of writing, or creating your business plan, or planning and saving for your life-changing around-the-world adventure every day will add up to great things much more quickly than you think. Instead of fantasizing abstractly about the life you could have had, take concrete steps toward building the life you want right now.

Don't know what that life is just yet? Or do you have a million ideas about what it might be? Take that half hour daily (or three times a week, or ten minutes a day) to dream about the changes you might make to achieve your next big step. Getting specific about your big, fat, hairy, audacious goals may be the toughest step of all. Then, once you have the beginnings of a vision, start using that set-aside time for action instead. As the plan starts to take shape, the amount of time you spend on it will naturally grow.

And then, if your goals shift—the novel doesn't get written, the big adventure doesn't manifest, and something else crops up organically in its place—that's okay. Better to discover that your vision still needs refining by experimentation than by betting the farm. You're still taking action, either toward your big next step or toward figuring out what it is. However you're spending that half hour a day, it's time very well spent. The fitness expert Todd Durkin, a former athlete who now trains high-performing franchise athletes like Drew Brees and Aaron Rodgers, calls it "blue sky" time: hours and minutes you set aside to consider, contemplate, and dream about what you want to do and where you want to go next. The sense of spaciousness and possibility that accompany those precious minutes and hours can be a powerful antidote to the feelings of limitation that many of us start to feel in our latter years.

Put simply, action is almost always the cure for apathy.

BRAINPOWER TIP #3: BREAK DOWN YOUR GOALS

> Nearly all rich, powerful people are not notably talented, educated, charming, or good-looking. They became rich and powerful by wanting to be rich and powerful. Your vision of where or who you want to be is the greatest asset you have. Without having a goal it's difficult to score.
>
> —PAUL ARDEN

By now you probably understand that we humans do best when we're working on a goal, ideally one that is challenging, fun, engaging, and exciting.

But how do you figure out what those goals might be? And how do you go about working on them? Let me answer that with a story about a guy I know.

Shannon Turley is the strength and conditioning coach for the Stanford University football team. But he's much, much more than that. Ask the average guy what a strength and conditioning coach does, and he'll tell you that he's the thick-necked knucklehead who loads barbells with huge weights and forces you to hoist them while he screams "ALL YOU!"

Turley is a different guy altogether. He stops short of being cerebral, but he's anything but a knucklehead.

Though most of the tools of the strength and conditioning trade are hewn from cold, hard iron, Turley will tell you that one of his most important weapons in getting his guys to step up and perform their best is the goal ladder. And it's printed on a sheet of paper.

When Turley took the job with Stanford a few years ago, he knew that everyone on the team wanted more or less the same thing: to stand out, be successful, win football games. But he found that wasn't enough. Goals, he knew, had to be specific. Superspecific. Micro, laser-pointer, on-the-money specific. They also had to be attainable. And there had to be a clear path to get there. So he created the "goal ladder," and he had each player fill one out.

Here's how a goal ladder works: At the top, you put one big, audacious goal. One that scares you a little. One that will take some effort to achieve. That's called your "outcome goal." For an athlete, maybe it would be "win the state championship." For a scientist, it might be "publish a groundbreaking study on animal behavior." For a lawyer, it might be "become a top-five earner in my firm." Whatever. It's the goal you dream about, and one you're not quite sure you can attain. Whatever goal you choose, that's your North Star: the direction you're going to point your ship, and the guiding principle of your career or business or creative life. That's the thing you'll want to keep your eye on.

An outcome goal might not be something you can control, entirely. Lots of factors go into a state championship, a groundbreaking study, and breaking the top five in earnings, and not all of them are up to you. That's okay. The outcome goal may be something you'll achieve, or it may not be. But it's something well worth shooting for. Something that fires you up. And, in truth, even falling a little short (being a top ten earner or making the playoffs), it will still be something to celebrate.

Below the top goal, you place two "performance goals." These are smaller goals that contribute to the bigger one. For the footballer, one might be "rush for one thousand yards this season." For the scientist, maybe it's "obtain grant money for three possible studies." For the lawyer, it might be "win two big cases and one smaller one this quarter."

At the base of the ladder, you place "process goals"—five for each performance goal. These are repeatable, daily (or weekly, or monthly) tasks that add up to the performance goals. They're things you have complete control over, and things *anyone* can do: "Get up at six and study the playbook daily." "Read an article a day on the mating behavior of marsupials." "Work on public speaking skills daily."

In turn, in an ideal world, these process goals would add up to the outcome goal at the top of the page. And voilà—you've climbed the goal ladder right to where you doubted you would be able to go. This means that the accomplishment of any huge goal is actually the result of simple, repeated, and repeatable tasks. It's a simple idea, but an incredibly powerful one. Don't let any get-rich-quick guru tell you any different.

Here is an example of my goal ladder that I developed when I decided to write this book:

OUTCOME GOAL

Write a bestselling book on men's health.

PERFORMANCE GOALS

Create most up-to-date, engaging, and inspiring text on the topic currently available.

Educate myself fully on the specific topics necessary to become a leading expert on the topic, able to promote book and discuss topics fluently and clearly.

PROCESS GOALS

1. Spend at least an hour a day reading peer-reviewed studies and popular articles on key topics.

2. Meet or consult at least one expert a week.

3. Discuss or email about key issues with trusted male friends in appropriate demographic at least once a week.

4. Test each idea by integrating at least *three* concepts or practices into my own life per week.

5. Write 500–1,500 words per weekday, one chapter per month.

6. Practice and sharpen discussion skills in all interactions on the topic.

Pretty simple, right? But also very powerful in how it focuses the small steps you need to take on a bigger goal or outcome. It reduces a pie-in-the-sky idea into manageable steps. If you can take those steps, you can achieve that big goal.

Take a minute (or five!) now, and write your own goal ladder for something you want to achieve this year.

Reminder: a goal ladder should be time-bound. You can have a goal ladder for a year, a quarter, or a month, as long as you choose a reasonable time frame. If it's too long, you won't do the actions you've committed to. Too short, and it may be unrealistic. Keep your goals as specific as possible and commit to the daily actions that will get you there. It's amazing what you can accomplish—and what obstacles you can overcome—when you go about it one tiny, deliberate step at a time. By contrast, when you're without a clear goal, you're disoriented. Your life lacks an organizing principle, and you're liable to be pulled off course by obstacles in your relationships, career, or by any of the thousands of competing demands that clamor for your attention all day, every day (until recently, I frequently had six screens ablaze in my office at any given time. When I'm not 100 percent on task, I can easily slip into wasting hours on any number of time-sucking websites.)

By the way—that Stanford football team? They went from a 1–11 team before Turley came to two Pac-12 championships just four years later. And it all started with those little pieces of paper.

YOU DON'T SUCK

Perception is reality.

Not long ago, my friend Laird Hamilton was approached by a young woman at his favorite coffee shop in Kauai (he's pretty hard to miss).

"This is such a coincidence," she gushed, "because I need your help! I've just started paddleboarding and I suck at it! What can I do to get better?"

"Here's your first lesson," Laird deadpanned. "You *don't* suck."

He got his coffee and strolled away.

The next day, he saw her again.

"I had the best day paddleboarding yesterday!" she gushed. "And you know what? You were right! I *don't* suck!"

Neither do you. So stop telling yourself, in a million tiny ways, that you do.

BRAINPOWER TIP #4: ACCEPT STRESS AS A GIVEN

As I mentioned in chapter 5, your autonomic nervous system works in seesaw fashion, ever toggling somewhere on the continuum between extreme arousal (fight-or-flight panic when the speeding cab nearly runs you down) and extreme relaxation (feed-and-breed relaxation as you catch rays on the beach). With the former, blood rushes to your extremities so you can use them as weapons. Reproductive and digestive functioning switch off. Pupils dilate. Tear and saliva secretion decreases. In extreme cases, your bladder relaxes and you lose hearing and peripheral vision. With the latter, your heart rate slows, your intestines and glands ramp up activity, and the sphincter muscles in your intestinal tract relax. The inner musculature of the penis may also relax, resulting in an erection.

Both these states serve important functions, of course: you need to get hyped-up to deal with real, physical challenges, and you need to chill out to rest, restore, digest, and reproduce.

The problem is that your autonomic nervous system evolved in an era when physical threats—in the form of predators, rival warring tribes, and errant rhinos—were much more common than they are today. When attack, assault, or mauling is a constant and ever-present threat, hypervigilance can be a very useful state to be able to achieve.

Relative to the threats we encounter now, though, the autonomic nervous system tends to be an overreactor. When the charging rhino is actually a jerk in a BMW in the adjacent lane, and the warring tribesman an ambulance-chasing lawyer, you don't need to fight or flee. You need to be able to stay calm and think clearly. But calm, rational thoughts are impaired when your sympathetic nervous system is on full alert.

And that's the predicament of the modern stressed-out middle-aged guy: our neuromuscular systems are primed and ready to fight off a tiger—but no tiger is forthcoming. We're all stressed-out with nowhere to go. And as a consequence, we aren't as focused or honed-in as we need to be. Our attention is diffused. We're too emotionally invested in the crisis all around us, and sometimes we explode, lashing out at others or falling into self-flagellation rather than focusing our attention to calmly and efficiently solve the problem at hand.

So what once helped keep your ancient ancestors alive long enough to spread a seed (a seed that would ultimately endure long enough to produce an ass-kicking New Primer like you) is now a liability. And it's not just a liability to your performance at work or your driving ability. Whereas the occasional burst of high stress, like what you get from exercise, can be beneficial, a chronically elevated stress response—the kind that many overworked and overcommitted men confront almost daily—can have many serious long-term health consequences, including many of the usual suspects:

- anxiety

- depression

- heart disease

- sleep problems

- weight gain

- memory and concentration impairment

Long-term stress, then, is an often-overlooked root cause of some of the most common ailments afflicting men over forty. And it's exacerbated by the fact that so many men are unable to talk about such feelings. I recently met the daredevil skydiver Felix Baumgartner, and we wound up chatting about the anxiety he faced when he was training for his world-record space jump. Here was a guy who has accomplished some of the most incredible feats in action sports. To me—and to most people who read about his spectacular feat—he is the ultimate alpha male. But because his public brand depends on his being completely fearless, he has to deal with his fears privately, out of the public gaze.

The line "men don't talk about their feelings" may sound like a 1950s sentiment, but it's one that still negatively affects us all. Many entrepreneurs who work and operate in high-stakes environments suffer under a similar gag rule, and they sometimes pay a very steep price for it: 34 percent of entrepreneurs admit to being "worried"; 45 percent say they are stressed. And, tragically, a few pay the ultimate price. Forty-nine-year-old banker Huibert Boumeester, fifty-four-year-old property tycoon Paul Castle, and fifty-one-year-old software innovator ReiJane Huai, all of whom had achieved enviable levels of success and wealth in their fields, took their own lives in recent years—most of them directly or indirectly because of work-related failures and challenges.

Toxic environmental and nutritional factors and a sedentary lifestyle can certainly exacerbate the classic health problems of the over-forty set. But stress—a chronic sense of being out of control of your own life—is a huge contributor to the midlife spiral that threatens to consume us, right around the time when we should be starting to thrive the most. And unfortunately, once it gets hold of you, the stress "weight gain and sleepless anxiety" cycle can be self-perpetuating—and very tough to escape.

Stress is out there, and it isn't going away for any of us. In 2012, 72 percent of survey respondents said their stress levels had increased or stayed the same over the previous five years, and 80 percent said their stress level had increased or stayed the same in the past year. Twenty percent of Americans report that their stress is "extreme" (eight, nine, or ten on a ten-point scale). The sources for all that stress probably sound familiar as well: 69 percent of respondents worried about money; 65 percent about work; 61 percent, the economy; 57 percent, family responsibilities; 56 percent, relationships; 52 percent, family health problems; and 51 percent, personal health concerns.

While we can certainly work on any or all of these areas—shoring up our health with diet and exercise, taking a good look at our personal budget to improve our financial outlook—it's hard to imagine a time when all of them will be 100 percent problem-free. Stress is always out there, in the background of all our lives in one shape or another. Many of us go through life thinking *if only I made x amount,* or *if only I had x job,* or *if only this or that problem would go away, all would be well.* But whether we reach those imaginary milestones or not, the stress doesn't go away. There's a temporary reduction in worry, and then we find new things to worry about, and new shoulda-coulda-woulda tapes play in our head.

So step one in conquering stress is to understand that life's pressures will almost always be with us. It's how we think about them—and the skill and finesse with which we ride those potentially stressful waves—that will spell the difference between whether we take a total wipeout into the surf or have a beautiful, smooth ride onto the shore.

BRAINPOWER TIP #5: SHIFT YOUR PERSPECTIVE

Reams of articles and books have been written on stress management, detailing how to reduce or eliminate it from your life, but I think many of them are wrongheaded. As I mentioned, long-term stress—for example, being on red alert for weeks or months at a time due to a high-pressure work project—is hell on your system. But short-term stress—those bursts of adrenaline we get in situations when we need to spring into action—is an essential part of life.

Men need stress to live. Every successful man in history—from Sir Isaac Newton to Steve Jobs—faced stressful situations in which the outcome was in doubt. Many of them faced extreme stress. It's part of what made them admirable.

And as evil as stress is made out to be in our culture, the fact is that we like stress. Most of our leisure activities—from skiing to mountain biking to watching sports to roller coasters to first-person-shooter video gaming—involve deliberately exposing ourselves to controlled, short-term forms of stress. For the most part, short-term stress is fun.

It's even good for you: studies indicate that people who have a robust short-term stress response—a pounding heart, a sweaty brow, rapid breathing—heal better after surgery or vaccination, and they may respond better to cancer treatment. Exercise and sex—activities that by now I hope I've convinced you are unequivocally good for you—both stimulate a hormonal response similar to what happens when you get charged by an angry pit bull.

One major key to conquering the bad kind of stress—the chronic version that keeps us up at night, distracts us from the things we enjoy most in life, and eats at our gut when we're trying to relax—is not so much to avoid it altogether but to reframe the way you think about it.

Sound abstract? Let me explain.

All of us have gone through busy periods in which our careers or families (or both) are demanding a lot of us: a big project is due, the boss is breathing down your neck, the house needs a new roof, your mother needs help at home, your son is starting in a playoff game, your wife is asking for a well-deserved night out. (A friend of mine recently joked that in times like these he feels as if every email in his inbox says "Dear Jack: Please do everything. Love, Everyone.")

Sometimes, those intense periods can make you want to crawl under a rock, leading you to drop the ball under pressure: the project is substandard, you miss the big game, and you fail to make dinner reservations—so you wind up in the doghouse, at work and at home. First you flail, then you fail. Other times, those intense periods have the opposite effect. Like a QB down by a field goal with seconds to play, you cowboy up and handle it, one task at a time, until you're on the other side of all that stress, with all your obligations signed, sealed, and delivered. And you feel like a superhero.

Interestingly, your ability to make it through those stressful situations with flying colors may hinge on how you *perceive* stress itself.

An eight-year study of thirty thousand adults of various ages found that people who experienced high stress and viewed stress as harmful to their health had a 43 percent higher risk of dying than others in the study. But people who experienced high stress—but did not consider stress harmful—had a much lower chance of dying. In fact, their risk of dying was even lower than those who experienced relatively little stress.

This is why I consider most of our beliefs about stress relief and the dangers of stress to be off base. *It may not be stress itself that's causing all the problems, but our* belief *that stress is inherently bad.*

A second study lends some support to this novel view. Two groups of adults were exposed to stressful situations: a math test with a judgmental instructor, and an impromptu public speaking assignment with a hostile audience. One group faced these situations cold. The second was told beforehand that the body's stress response was beneficial in high-pressure situations—a physiological marshalling of forces that helped them meet the challenges with which they were confronted.

Both groups experienced the pounding heart, shortness of breath, and sweaty palms we associate with stress. But the cardiovascular response to these situations was markedly different in the two groups. The blood vessels in the group that went into the stressful situations cold constricted strongly, a response that, coupled with a rapid heart, can lead to cardiac disease over time. By contrast, the blood vessels in the group that was given the "stress is good" pep talk dilated—a physiological response similar to what we experience in moments of joy or courage. Over many years, the difference between these two responses to stress—one detrimental, the other salutary—can spell the difference between dying at a younger age and living to a ripe old age (with many stories to tell of the heart-pounding adventures you've undergone in your long, colorful life).

So aside from finding ways to avoid chronic stress, simply thinking of your short-term stress response as your body helping you rise to the demands of a challenging situation can mitigate the damage that stress can cause. And now that you've heard about it, remind yourself of it whenever you get stressed. You may even thank your body for its efforts to protect you and help you perform optimally. The outward signs of stress may remain—maybe your hands will get clammy, maybe your heart will pound—but inside, you'll be healthier for it.

FIND YOUR "OPTIMAL STRESS ZONE"

Stress has the power to make you great—and to hobble you with anxiety and fear. How do you find that optimal place where stress focuses you and brings out the best? The key appears to be to take on your stressful activity in controlled waves, interspersed with more relaxing, mellowing-out activities.

Say you have a huge report due in six hours. Redlining for the full 360 minutes won't bring out your best work, suggests new research by Dr. Herbert Benson of the Mind/Body Institute in Chestnut Hill, Massachusetts. Instead, work until you feel that "overwhelmed" sensation just start to crest. Then, take a break and do something that chills you out. Draw a picture, meditate, do some push-ups, play your guitar, run around the block, chat about irrelevant things.

When you do that abrupt U-turn just before the full swan-dive-out-the-boardroom-window panic attack, a biochemical reaction kicks in and leads to new creativity and higher performance that can last for some time.

Of course, it's best not to be in a situation in which you have just six hours to crank out a report. But on those occasions when you do, you can reach new heights of performance under stress by learning to surf the wave of your natural stress response.

BRAINPOWER TIP #6: CONNECT

> You are the average of the five people you spend the most time with.
>
> —JIM ROHN

You've heard it before: *man is a social animal*. And it's the truth. We like to think we're independent, up-by-the-bootstraps, self-reliant John Wayne types, never asking for a free lunch. But it ain't so: not one of us would have made it much past a few hours old without all kinds of help from the adults around us. Unlike, say, sharks, whose mothers swim blithely away after giving birth, humans are born helpless. We need nurturing, feeding, and educating for many years before we can hope to survive on our own.

But we need other people beyond infancy. In Paleolithic times, man's capacity to cooperate with other men—to work together to build shelters, bring down large prey, grow food, travel long distances, and raise and protect children—was what allowed him to survive, thrive, and eventually become the dominant species on earth (it certainly wasn't his physical strength, speed, or acute senses, all of which were laughable when compared with many other competing species). It's part of what makes us who we are.

News flash: as a gender, we men aren't that great at connecting with others. We're terrible at reaching out to other people when we're in a time of need. Or, equally, when someone else is in need. We've seen one too many movies and TV shows propagating the lone, strong, capable hero myth, and we've swallowed it hook, line, and sinker.

Successful men, in particular, are prone to the "lone wolf" syndrome. "Alpha males," who have often built their livelihoods on being independent-minded leaders and appearing fearless and decisive to others, may hesitate to open up for fear of appearing weak; no one wants to be the "beta male." As a result, they've fallen out of the practice of opening up, and they wind up perpetuating their own isolation.

Consider the "male deficit model," a sociological theory based on thirty years of data on friendship and relationships. According to this theory—which has its roots in a 1982 UCLA study on the differences between male and female relationships—our friendships are far less intimate than women's. We compete with our friends more, and report lower satisfaction with our relationships with friends. And the more we adhere to antiquated ideas of manhood—the strong, silent approach—the worse off our friendships are.

Missing out on friendship has more serious consequences than you might think. Loneliness reduces cognition and motor function, and it increases stress hormones and perhaps even chronic inflammation. According to a recent review study encompassing over a quarter-million test subjects, loneliness is just as bad for your health as smoking fifteen cigarettes a day, or alcohol addiction, or not exercising. It's twice as bad for you as being obese.

On the flip side, research suggests that having strong social connections is a major factor in living a long, happy life, perhaps equal to eating a good diet, getting proper exercise, and maintaining healthy sleep habits. In fact, a single good friend can increase your life expectancy by ten years. According to the "Blue Zones" research, having strong social connections is one of the key factors in extraordinary longevity. One 2010 study even found that strong social ties are the number one predictor of survival among cancer patients.

Bad news for men who want to connect socially with other men: poker nights, bowling leagues, and nights out with the guys are slowly becoming things of the past. Even if our dads were involved in such things, it's more and more unlikely that we are. According to a longitudinal study, the median number of people in a "network of confidants" (tight groups of intimate friends) decreased from 2.94 to 2.08 people from 1985 to 2004. Twenty-five percent of Americans said they had no one to talk to at all in 2004. For most of us, family has replaced community. And as admirable as that may seem, while friendships add measurable years to your life, family relationships have a negligible effect on longevity.

So having no friends is bad for you—inside and out—and having strong friendships can have many health benefits, and might even save you from cancer. But how many of these friends do you need for the benefits to kick in?

Since you're a guy, I'll get down to brass tacks for you: you need three *real* friends.

Dr. Robin Dunbar, an anthropologist at Oxford and an expert on human societies, has found that most people are capable of maintaining stable relationships with about 150 people. Ten to fifteen of them will be members of a "sympathy group," and three to five will be close friends who can be relied on in times of trouble. Four-o'clock-in-the-morning friends. Guys who would visit you in the hospital if you needed them to. Guys who would bail you out of jail. Guys you can confide in.

When thinking about the state of your friendships, consider the following:

- Who are the friends who would stick by you if you didn't have the job you have, the money you have, or the wife or partner you have? Which of the people you know are stand-up enough to be there for you no matter what?

- Conversely, are you a good enough friend to be there for the people you know as well? Have you taken such steps for anyone outside your inner circle? How often do you take steps to make someone feel supported and important?

You probably have many *acquaintances*—from work, through your wife's friends or your kids' school—with whom you'd probably enjoy spending some time outside of the office or school parking lot. If, like so many other men, you're lacking in the friend department, then proactively cultivate those relationships. Go get coffee or a beer, shoot some hoops, go surfing or play tennis. Guys do well with structured, repeated, time-bound activities, and many men find their closest friends in formal men's groups dedicated specifically to deepening men's connections with one another. Whether or not that's your thing personally, a strong and ongoing connection to your friends is one of the most essential components in your long-term health and well-being—so find a way to make those connections.

During the summer, I often get together for workouts with a group that includes many super accomplished alpha males, among them the surfing star Laird Hamilton, the fitness icon Darin Olien, and überfit character actor John C. McGinley, as well as producers and directors of some of the world's major blockbuster movies. Laird outlines the activities for the morning—usually a punishing combination of bodyweight strength moves, swim training, core exercises, and ice water immersion. It's always incredibly challenging, but it's also richly rewarding—not only because the workout is so tough, but also because being in the presence of so many successful guys who all share similar values is inspiring. Everyone bonds over the challenges of the workouts, and we all celebrate the fitness and mental breakthroughs we individually make. We're also aware of the personal challenges each of us faces—in business, career, family, and relationships—and, between sets and after the workout, we check in with each other about how our lives are going.

Like Laird, all of these men are at the top of their field: high performers who strive for excellence in every area of their lives. Their company helps keep me sharp, always pushing me to do more in my businesses, career, and life—rather like a tennis player playing up to the level of his competition. If I spent a lot of time with less successful men, I imagine the opposite would happen, just as it does when I play tennis against players who are less skilled than I am: my own game suffers. Even when your life is on track, other successful people can inspire you, show you what's possible, and introduce novel approaches to business, career, and family that may not have occurred to you. Those are the people you want to surround yourself with: the guys who help you play up a level.

It also helps that many of these guys are younger than I am. It keeps me feeling sharp and relevant and on top of things. And there's no better feeling, as a guy in his fifties, than keeping up with guys who are ten and twenty years younger.

As I write this, I'm four weeks out from a three-day hike along a section of the John Muir Trail, a rugged 220-mile path along the backbone of the High Sierras in California, which concludes with an ascent up Mount Whitney, the highest summit in the contiguous United States. My climbing partners: two guys in their twenties.

Most men my age would be worried that they'd be the weak link in such a group, and would thus beg off. I'm expecting to be inspired—and hopefully to inspire them, too—by showing them what thirty-five years of fitness training can do for you when you're pushing hard to the summit of a fourteen-thousand-foot mountain. I intend to look for more challenges with vital, inspiring people for the rest of my life: projects that force me to challenge myself and call on reserves of energy and tenacity that I didn't know I had.

The right people (and they're often younger people) can allow you to expect more out of yourself—and ultimately to get more out of yourself. Sadly, the opposite can be true as well: Maria and I recently met a very fit and active seventy-year-old man and his vivacious sixty-five-year-old wife who said that many of their old friends were slowing down due to obesity, joint pain, and simple resignation. Their less-healthy friends seemed to feel no desire to travel or experience new things, right when this couple had started to dive in—and they felt this was personally slowing them down as a result. The couple told us they were in the process of redefining these relationships for that very reason: they didn't want their friends to hold them back in life.

If you're hesitant about cultivating relationships with people who are younger than you, remember that you have something to offer them as well. The young guys in Laird's group appreciate the informal mentoring that naturally occurs when younger and older guys begin talking about shared interests, goals, and ambitions. When I was living my surfer lifestyle on the Gold Coast, I had the benefit of many older mentors who helped me along in both my academic and business lives. I wouldn't be where I am today without the help of guys who took the time and energy to guide me, and now I'm happy to pay it forward.

I'm grateful and fortunate to have these guys in my life—it's one of the reasons I travel an hour and a half from Newport Beach to Malibu to train with them. I feel like my connection with them, and the other half dozen or so close friends with whom I stay in touch regularly, represents a new branching out in my life. I've gone through phases in which I've been extremely focused on my career, and whittled my social circle down substantially. My career flourished during those times, but looking back I know I felt isolated. My sense of happiness and value as a man rose or fell with the fluctuations of my stock portfolio. Maria was always her supportive self, of course, but without other men to connect to, who shared similar pressures and aspirations, my life was much more limited. In the last few years, I've placed a much higher priority on social connections, and I've been much happier for it.

Some men find similar solace in more official male-only or largely male groups. The YPO—Young Presidents' Organization—caters to the specific concerns of business leaders. Because many of the members are well known, the organization operates under a code of complete silence, kind of like *Fight Club*: what gets discussed at the meetings stays at the meetings. As a result, its members feel safe about opening up, and lots of good truth-telling occurs when its members get together. Not everyone is a young president, of course, but many such groups are out there, each dealing with a different type of men's issue. And if, like most men, you lack a lot of support from other guys, these groups are well worth exploring.

One final, interesting physiological fact about social connection: it's a potent, automatic stress reliever. Oxytocin, sometimes known as the "cuddle hormone" because mothers secrete it when they nurse, is also secreted by both men and women when they interact socially. It's associated with greater empathy and feelings of connection.

The kicker, though, is that it's also released during times of stress: when we're under intense pressure, our bodies signal us to reach out to others, and connect with them. This may be nature's way of telling us to work together when times are tough. When normal citizens risk their lives to come to the aid of complete strangers during large-scale disasters, that may be the biological imperative of oxytocin: nature telling us to reach out and help others.

But we don't need to wait for an emergency to take advantage of this physiological urge. If you're stressed-out, connect with someone. If possible, help someone. Better yet, make volunteering in some capacity a regular part of your life. Your body is asking for it.

BRAINPOWER TIP #7: MEDITATE

> What we think of as "normal" aging in our society is not really normal. It's the psychopathology of a person who is totally stressed-out. My research indicates that meditating slows cell death, lowering your "biological age," which dictates how you look and feel. It allows the body to heal itself. Start with five minutes every morning.
>
> —DEEPAK CHOPRA, MD

In the last few years, meditation has been making its way, gradually, from the realm of the Buddhist, the hippie, and the yogi (and the hipster versions of all three) into the mainstream.

Hugh Jackman meditates. So do Rupert Murdoch, Bill Ford, Oprah Winfrey, David Lynch, Ray Dalio, Paul McCartney, and Jerry Seinfeld. Execs at Apple, Facebook, Nike, Google, and AOL are all promoting the practice in-house.

It's all for a very good reason, and if you're not on the meditation bandwagon right now, it's time you considered it.

Why?

Meditation, research has shown, increases gray-matter density in areas of the brain associated with learning, memory, attention, and empathy. An article in the *Journal of Neuroscience* recently reported that in people who experience discomfort, meditation can reduce pain intensity by 40 percent.

Personally, though, I meditate for a much simpler reason: It quiets the *noise*.

"Mental noise," it turns out, may be one of our biggest obstacles to success. The National Science Foundation tells us that the average person has fifty thousand distinct thoughts per day. High-performers, however, have just eighteen thousand.

It's the opposite of what we'd expect, isn't it? We think that high-performers must be popping with ideas 24-7, and lesser mortals are slower thinkers. But if you look deeper, it makes sense. High-functioning people have less noise, less distraction, less self-sabotaging chatter, and more focus and concentration on their goals. The scattered brain constantly offers up options, wanting us to *choose something*; the focused, streamlined brain makes its choices more efficiently. Like a good coach or brilliant athlete, it's in action mode. No time for too much naval-gazing.

You've probably had experiences that bear this out. When you're stressed, the mind seems to race, desperately trying to come up with a plan. When you're calm, your thoughts are clear, quiet, streamlined. The brain, says the performance coach Todd Herman, is naturally *teleological*—goal seeking—and when there is no goal, it races around like an overeager puppy looking for one.

Unfortunately, you burn a lot of energy this way.

Sometimes my "days off" are among the most stressful days of the week. My body might be relaxing or doing something enjoyable, but I can't let go of some issue—personal, professional, financial. My mind keeps coming back to it, sniffing around the issue or just reminding me that it's there and I haven't dealt with it. At the end of the day I'm often more stressed-out and exhausted than if I'd spent the day working.

One of the best tools for distilling all the mind chatter—and one I've only recently discovered—is meditation. Sitting quietly. Eyes closed. Breathing. And thinking about . . . nothing.

Sounds simple, right? Yet people spend their whole lives perfecting this simple act. Stilling the mind. Focusing on the nothingness.

Many men (Westerners, in particular) find meditating extremely uncomfortable at first. Sitting (or standing, or lying completely still), without watching TV, listening to music, or intending to go to sleep, is an unusual endeavor for time-constrained guys in this age of constant intake and output of information. Why would I just sit still when I could be answering email, checking Facebook or Instagram, or texting one of my three hundred contacts?

The first time you try it, you'll probably be astounded at the thoughts that race through your mind, and the frantic pace at which they come. Crazy, insane ideas, funny images, anxiety-producing scenarios. That's your "monkey mind" or "untamed horse" doing its dance, trying to come up with ideas to divert your attention from simply *being*. Over time, probably in your first five-minute session, you'll find a small place, perhaps by accident, where you're not thinking. The monkey stops. Life, for a moment, seems simple. You accept it. You're at peace.

It will last about one second, and you might not even notice it. But that's what you want to build on. Really good meditators can stay there for hours. But even when you don't pull off that nirvana state (and I myself rarely achieve it for very long), you'll still get benefits, among them:

- reduced blood pressure
- reduced tension-related pain (tension headaches, ulcers, insomnia, muscle and joint problems)
- reduced negative emotions
- decreased anxiety and stress
- increased mood-boosting serotonin
- increased immunity
- increased energy
- better healing
- improved emotional stability and mental clarity
- improved creativity and happiness

That all sounds pretty awesome, right?

Some thoughts on how to meditate: You'll see some longtime meditators sitting *seiza* (in a kneeling position) with their eyes closed, chanting or contemplating a candle or a flower. Others practice slow movements, like tai chi, qi gong, or yoga, while meditating. I encourage you to try all of these practices, and I know that the more you meditate, the more benefits you will receive. But also remember that you don't need to make it the center of your life. You can meditate virtually anywhere or anytime: waiting at a stoplight, standing in a grocery line, riding the subway. You can meditate taking a walk. The keys to a satisfying meditation are:

- **Focusing your attention** on your breath, a mantra, or some external, beautiful, inspiring object. This allows your thoughts to become clearer and quieter.

- **Relaxing your breath,** allowing your diaphragm to fully relax and expand your lungs. Don't push too much for a deep breath—let the air come in and out naturally and allow it to slow as you relax more deeply. Remember to feel the rise and fall of your stomach—not your chest. If all that's rising and falling is your chest, then you are not getting the full benefit of the breath—it's constricted, most likely due to stress.

- **Quieting down.** Again—you can meditate anywhere, and practiced meditators can find a place of inner calm even amid chaos and extreme stress. In his book *Dharma in Hell,* the Zen teacher Fleet Maull talks about finding a place of inner calm while sitting on a bunk in a prison cell where he spent fourteen years with convicted murderers, armed robbers, and sex offenders around every corner. But too many noisy distractions can pull your attention outward, especially when you're first beginning. Finding a quiet place is ideal.

- **Getting comfortable.** Don't assume you have to sit in any particular way to meditate "correctly": sit, stand, lie down, kneel, and shift when you need to. You can't focus when you're uncomfortable.

A little bit about my personal practice: I attend the Shambhala Temple in Orange County for weekly meditation, and I follow Sakyong Mipham Rinpoche, whose book *Turning the Mind into an Ally* is a must-read for people wanting to go deep into meditation.

My personal meditation practice consists of a minimum of fifteen minutes, morning and night, following this template:

- **Getting comfortable** on my meditation pillow. I sit upright, legs crossed and hands on my knees, palms up. My posture is straight, which allows the breath to flow naturally. My mouth and jaw are relaxed, so breath can flow easily. My eyes are slightly closed and fixed on a point about two feet in front of me.

- **Focusing on my breath.** Like an ocean wave, the natural in-and-out flow of breath can be very soothing. But you can't focus on it too intensely—or your mind will spin out into too many concrete thoughts. Nor can you be too relaxed, or your mind will get fuzzy. Breathe normally but always be conscious of the breath.

- **Allowing thoughts to come and go.** Thoughts will constantly come up—even the best meditators cannot avoid this. The trick, if such a thing can be said to exist in meditation, is to let those thoughts come and go. Recognize when they do and gently steer your attention back to your breath, allowing the thoughts to just float by, like a cloud.

- **Being gentle.** Meditation teaches you to be easy with yourself. So many self-improvement programs ask that you become a strenuous, effortful version of yourself. They suggest that you can do anything you want if you want it badly enough, work hard enough, focus more intensely on your goals. This is good counsel in certain contexts, but in meditation you do none of those things; instead, you allow yourself to simply breathe and be—rather than forcing yourself, out of habit, into action.

- **Bringing the mind back to the breath.** Each time you recognize that your mind has wandered away from the breath, and you gently return to it, your mind gets a little bit stronger. It's like a repetition in the weight room. You're building and strengthening a skill. So don't judge or chastise yourself for having irrelevant thoughts any more than you'd judge a barbell for falling to the floor when you drop it.

Keep that up for fifteen minutes, twice a day, and you'll be on the path toward wisdom and compassion (not to over-promise or anything).

Meditation (which I just mistyped as "medication"—an interesting Freudian slip of the fingers!) has come to feel more and more profound to me as I've gotten older. I meditate in the morning as a way of staving off the frantic "ready, set, GO!" mentality that can descend on anyone who's focused on taking big steps and living to his potential in the world. I'll meditate for ten to fifteen minutes before bed as a way of slowing down and clearing out the mental clutter before I shut down for the night. And I'll do more whenever I get a moment.

It's a life-changer.

BRAINPOWER TIP #8: PRACTICE HAPPINESS HYGIENE

> The goal is not to be better than the other man, but your previous self.
>
> —DALAI LAMA XIV

> Over time our society's notion of success has been reduced to money and power. In fact, at this point, success, money, and power have practically become synonymous in the minds of many. This idea of success can work—or at least appear to work—in the short term. But over the long term, money and power by themselves are like a two-legged stool—you can balance on them for a while, but eventually you're going to topple over.
>
> —ARIANNA HUFFINGTON

The broad strokes of most men's life plans go something like this:

1. Go to school.
2. Get a job.
3. Marry a beautiful partner.
4. Get a more important job.
5. Amass wealth and success.
6. Repeat steps 4–5 until retirement or death.

Notice how *enjoyment* is nowhere in this list? The number one concern of many of our important life choices, whether we think about it or not, is very often money. The prospect of spending any significant amount of time doing anything we truly enjoy, by contrast, is a far-off, abstract dream.

So the question as to why we're unhappy actually has a pretty obvious answer. Quite simply, we're unhappy because we don't structure our lives around activities that make us happy. Instead, we structure them around activities that make us *money*.

And unhappy we are: Suicides among men in midlife have jumped 50 percent in the last fifteen years. It's the biggest jump seen in any demographic in recent times—male, female, young, middle-aged, or older.

Scientists don't really know why so many men our age are so desperately unhappy, but I have a guess: it comes from too much comparing—and from the ubiquity of social networks.

To start, we compare our life as it is with the life we expected we would have at this age. And I don't care how rich, happily married, impressively credentialed, or well-connected you are—there's always a gap. In most cases, a pretty big one.

We also compare ourselves with each other. If it seems as though Mr. Jones down the street is happier, richer, fitter, or whatever-er than we are, we feel like we're not measuring up. And most of what we see, hear, and read about in popular media every day is about spectacular achievers at their most spectacular: this or that movie star, athlete, or newly minted Internet billionaire.

Social media hasn't made things any easier. On Facebook (and Instagram, and everywhere else online), all we see are the successes of our "friends" and the highlights of their lives. The picture painted by social media is such that everybody's life is perfect, full of perfect holidays, friends, partners, and life. It's Elysium. And that's what we compare ourselves with as well.

Aspirations are important, and we all have idols. But when we constantly berate ourselves for not being absolutely perfect in every department, we'll always come up short. And that, I think, is our undoing on the happiness front.

I'll also add that working harder—putting in longer hours, and struggling to become a more efficient, strenuously perfect version of ourselves—rarely works either. It doesn't get us closer to this elusive state called "happiness."

So if obsessively comparing ourselves with others, and single-mindedly pursuing materialistic goals won't make us happier, what does?

The answer is more obvious than you think: *doing things you love.*

Do you love skiing? Put your skiing dates in your calendar and treat them like real appointments you can't break. Running? Block off three days a week for a run at lunch so everyone in your office knows you aren't taking appointments. Revel in your run and go back to work recharged and ready for more.

This is different from the Big Rocks advice earlier in this book. This is more like "happiness hygiene" (a phrase I think I just invented): repeated activities you do largely because they maintain your mood and outlook.

Quite logically, the daily practice of things that make you happy will go a long way toward actually making you happy—much more so than delaying happiness to some far-off time when all bills are paid and all kids are through school. Many of us have learned the "delay of gratification" lesson too well, so that we just keep putting it off till we're dead.

Now that you're over forty, this is the time to get going on those long-delayed desires, interests, and aspirations. Quit waiting.

And when you're making big life choices—like where to live or what job to take—make day-to-day enjoyment a game-changing part of the equation. Moving to Boise, Idaho, to be a VP of a potato-peeling company may be a prestigious and high-paying leap from where you are now, but unless you love the smell of potatoes, the Western climate and countryside, and the day-to-day activities of your prospective job, turn it down—no matter the money, no matter the perks, no matter how good it seems in the abstract. Day-to-day reality, much more so than some abstract idea ("I'm making a difference"; "I'm an executive vice president"), is what has the biggest influence on happiness.

The best big-picture life goal and the bottom-line key to happiness is finding work that combines meaning and enjoyment. You'll note that money is nowhere in that equation. So make changes, big and small, that allow you to do the things you love often.

TRAIN YOUR MEMORY

How many times have you showed up at work on a Monday and been asked "How was your weekend?" only to be unable to recall a single thing from the previous two days? If you're like most people, the answer is "all the time."

You're not losing your mind, you're just not in the habit of recalling things. You have experiences and they pass through you without sticking. For some parts of our lives, this may be a good thing. If you had to give 100 percent focus to every little action you do, from brushing your teeth to driving to work, you'd miss out on a lot of brainless, dreamy contemplation time.

But certain things—your wife's birthday and your day's appointment schedule, for example—are well worth remembering. Perhaps even more important, you don't want to forget those little inspirations you have at random times—in the shower, on a run or a bike ride—throughout the day. Those little inklings can eventually form the foundation of a new direction in your life. They're little imps whispering in your ear, urging you toward a better version of yourself.

Most of us have a fear of losing our memory—and with the prevalence of Alzheimer's disease and dementia among older men, this fear is understandable. As the film *Total Recall* suggests, the aggregate of your memories constitutes who you are in many ways. The mental storehouse of your remembered experiences is what makes up your identity. So, even the smallest indication that you're losing your grip on those fragile images and sound bites can be unsettling indeed.

Like virtually anything else, though, you can train your memory. Here's how:

PRACTICE TOTAL RECALL

Every night before you fall asleep, go through your day, one action at a time. What time did you wake up? What did you do first? What did you eat? Where did you go? Whom did you talk to? Remember in as much detail as possible—right down to the name of the barista who got your coffee at Starbucks. After you've done this for a few days, try recalling two days before, then three, four, and so on.

LEARN NEW STUFF

Crossword puzzles are one clichéd way of staying mentally sharp, but there are many, many others—most of which involve learning or refining a skill. Learning a new language or a new song on a musical instrument, or memorizing text, poetry, or inspirational quotes are all great ways to strengthen your memory. I'd also urge you to read as broadly as you can and never stop learning. At present, I have about thirty active monthly subscriptions, including such diverse publications as *Popular Mechanics*, *National Geographic*, *Psychology Today*, and *Scientific American*.

In addition, new physical experiences and skills translate into more synaptic connections. This is part of the reason I vary my workouts so much—it keeps my brain healthy and young by focusing on new moves and techniques. It's also why I took up flying lessons.

Bottom line: keep busy—mentally and physically—to stay sharp.

WRITE STUFF DOWN

The simple act of writing things down is incredibly powerful. The walls of my office in Newport Beach are covered, virtually floor to ceiling, with whiteboard paint. I love being able to jot things down, to get my thoughts out into a visible form. I keep notepads everywhere for this same reason, and frequently use the recorder function, the Notes app, and Siri on my iPhone to get my ideas down. I've been known to jump out of the shower to get something down on paper before stepping back in to finish washing up. It's scary, but sometimes you can lose a thought in the time it takes to get to a pen and paper!

What you write down is what you'll remember, act on, do, and realize. Of course, writing also makes you translate a vague inkling into language you understand, which is the first step to getting it done. And once you've written it, you can release it into the universe. It's on the list, so you don't have to keep it in your brain.

One final tool I love: wunderlist.com. It allows you to make lists (I'm obsessed with lists) that you can share with collaborators—and update them constantly. I highly recommend it.

PAY ATTENTION

According to research, memory is driven by adrenaline. Those events in our lives that excite us—getting married, having a child, taking your company public—tend to be driven into our memories more completely. That's part of why you don't remember a boring weekend. So part of remembering is being present. It means slowing down the noise in your head long enough to notice things like the new flowers in the neighbor's yard as you get into your car to drive to work. Attention is a hidden, powerful discipline, and it's a key to keeping the memory sharp.

BRAINPOWER TIP #9: DEFRY YOUR BRAIN

In some ways, our dads had it easy. When they got home from work, they were *home*. If they didn't bring a briefcase full of documents back from the office, work would have to wait until tomorrow. If they needed a piece of information from the library or a six-month-old newspaper, they—or someone, anyway—had to go get it. And they had to wait. They didn't have the option to do anything from anywhere, all the time.

That sounds medieval in today's world, of course, where virtually everything we need, short of the most specialized knowledge and firsthand experience, is a few clicks away. But this linear ordering of information and step-by-step process forced the men of our dads' generation to work at what might be called an analog pace. It allowed them to think clearly, one project, one event, one sentence at a time.

I know I'm waxing nostalgic about the glories of the good old days here (it's an occupational hazard for men over fifty), but one major challenge of the digital age is that everything appears to have an equal priority, from the reminder that our quarterly taxes are due (truly urgent) to our daughter's text asking if she can go out to dinner with a friend next Friday (less so) to the ping from our YouTube cat-video subscription channel (utterly insignificant). But in digital land, each piece of incoming information appears to hold the same sway. How often do you receive emails with "URGENT" in the subject line—which then turn out to be about as urgent as last year's box scores? I rest my case.

When I first set up my Newport Beach office, I was excited to have the space for six big computer screens, where I'd have six projects going at once. I figured I'd be more productive than ever. My office was like a NASA command center.

Guess what? The opposite happened. I *started* tons of things. But I *finished* almost none of them.

It was too overwhelming. Facebook pings. *Huffington Post* articles. Emails. I'd arrive at the office with six important items on my to-do list, and immediately twenty others would pop up to overtake them. Everything was in my face, 24-7, and it was so overwhelming that it was impossible to connect with what was truly important to me. I was always on the defensive, besieged with the world's requests of me—and the constant seduction of the digital sphere.

A University of Sussex study suggests that there may well be a physiological reason for my feelings. Multiscreening, the study found, actually causes brain damage—a loss of gray matter in the anterior cingulate cortex, an area in the brain responsible for regulating emotions, decision-making, impulse control, and reasoning. Numerous other studies have linked high computer and mobile device use with depression, insomnia, loss of empathy, and an inability to relate to people one-on-one. In my case, I started to feel that I was losing the ability to focus on tasks—and now I realize why.

Tony Robbins has written about four types or dimensions of tasks. They are categorized as:

1. Not *urgent*, and not *important*.

2. *Urgent*, but not *important*.

3. *Important* and *urgent*.

4. *Important*, but not *urgent*.

The first is the dimension of *distraction*: Playing video games. Watching TV. Facebook. Porn. Time-wasting.

The second is the dimension of *delusion*: you decide you need to get to the movie right on time, or send a text at this instant, so you literally risk your life—or at least a stiff fine—speeding to get to the theater or texting behind the wheel.

The third is the dimension of *demand*: you're working on something significant under a strict and intense deadline. A trial that could save or lose someone money or freedom. A report that could alter the course of a company. Many work environments are set up to operate largely in this third dimension—*everything* is important, and it needs to have been done yesterday. I've worked in environments like this before. It's the prime heart-attack dimension: you're hunkered down, running on all cylinders, never able to catch your breath.

TAKE A DIGITAL DETOX

I've mentioned this elsewhere in the book, but it's an essential practice that deserves another reminder: choose times during the day that are sacred, when you can't be reached digitally. That means severing the umbilical-like connection to your computer, iPad, and, yes, your smartphone.

Big deal, you say? Try it. Many guys have a serious problem with it, and they immediately come up with rationalizations like "I need to know where my kids are!"

You don't, actually. Not 24-7.

Checking texts, emails, box scores, the stock market, Facebook, and so on is a tic, a crutch, a kind of addiction—and most of us are hooked, to some extent. You never needed round-the-clock access to this kind of information before your smartphone existed, and you don't need it now.

I think of my iPhone as a devil in my pocket. I try to be "good," by taking a hike, talking with my wife, working on important projects, but I always know that a funny video or an interesting news story is just a click away. I recently took a hike with a very single male friend of mine who spent the whole time on Tinder. We were in the middle of nowhere, on a mountaintop. He logged on, broadcasting to the world that he was available and interested. Within seconds, twelve women indicated that they were up for hooking up with him. Right then, right there. A dozen in-the-flesh hookups were just a swipe away.

Those are the kinds of temptations that are available to us at all times—and I can only imagine how this will evolve a few years from now.

Don't get me wrong, I love technology. But more and more, the most intimate and foundational interactions of our lives are mediated by technology, and, convenient as that can be, it's not the real thing. Unplugging multiple times a day, and ideally for one full day per week, is essential to maintaining perspective and real connection with the real world. To separate yourself from the incessant, invasive clamor of technology, spend time in nature—where the stillness and majesty of trees, water, stones, earth, and sky remind you of your roots and your connection to something much more eternal and vast than the blurry, insubstantial, blink-and-it's-gone world of ones and zeros.

We all spend time in these first three dimensions, but none of them is overly satisfying. The "sweet spot," Robbins argues, is the fourth dimension—the dimension of *fulfillment*. That's where you're working on something significant, but you're not under a crazy deadline. There's time and space to consider it. It's your long-term big project. It's your exercise program. It's preparing your next healthy meal. It's thinking about your long-term plans with your spouse. It's your true North Star.

Most of us spend the majority of our time in the "demand" and "delusion" dimensions and reward ourselves, after a long, rat-racey day, with some distraction. We keep meaning to get to the fulfillment stuff, but it never materializes. We "to-do list" ourselves right out of our biggest dreams and aspirations.

Want to defry your brain? Rejigger your day to make the dimension of fulfillment more of a priority. I've already suggested that you meditate and exercise early in the day, and that you carve out time for the contemplation of bigger projects and life dreams. How else can you flip the ordering of things to assert more control, and spend more time in the fulfillment zone?

Hit that fourth dimension more often, and you're sure to be on target with your actual purpose, and the stuff that really matters to you.

Oh—and I've gotten rid of all but two of those screens in my office. I consider that progress toward fulfillment.

BRAINPOWER TIP #10: SLEEP YOURSELF BETTER, SMARTER, FASTER

Let's say you're forty-five years old and that you sleep an average of seven hours a night. Maybe that's wishful thinking, but remember that you probably slept almost twice that for the first few years of your life. At forty-five, you've been alive about 16,425 days—and you've slept for 4,790 of them—the equivalent of over *thirteen years*.

Consider what a huge chunk of time that is. This very day you could start from scratch on virtually any activity your health and talents would allow and could be world-class at it in thirteen years if you applied yourself. If you have kids, consider what stage of life they'll be at in thirteen years compared with now. It's a precious, powerful, life-changing chunk of time. And you've already invested that amount of time in sleep, and will hopefully invest at least as much again before you pack it in, bringing your total time spent snoozing to well above the quarter-century mark. Whoa.

Sleep is mysterious thing. After millennia of speculation and research, no one really knows why we need it, just that we do—desperately. Animals deprived of sleep lose immune function and die after only a few weeks, and cognitive and physical function decline measurably after just one night of poor sleep.

So did we evolve to stay still, quiet, and out of harm's way when predators—and toe-stubbing rocks and logs—were out in the dark, seeking to do us harm? Does sleep help us conserve energy, and therefore precious resources? (Consider those 2:00 a.m. munchies when you're pulling an all-nighter.)

One theory that has gained traction in recent years is that we need sleep to restore function. Muscle growth, tissue repair, growth hormone release, and protein synthesis all happen primarily while you're snoozing. Cognitive function is also affected by sleep. During wakefulness, cell activity in the brain produces a by-product called adenosine, which builds up gradually throughout the day and is cleared at night. Adenosine buildup may be one signal for drowsiness.

The newest thought about why we need sleep is that it allows our brains to shift and grow. If you've ever woken up with an obvious solution to what felt the night before like an insurmountable problem, you've experienced this firsthand. Sleep signals the brain to restructure and reorganize, to build new neural connections and new associations. It can be difficult for us hard-charging, problem-solving guys to understand, but sometimes the best way to fix a problem is to back off it for a little while, because in a very real, tangible sense, sleep makes you better.

According to statistics reported by the Centers for Disease Control and Prevention, about 30 to 40 percent of men and women get fewer than seven hours of sleep per night. About one-third of adults unintentionally fell asleep during the day over the past thirty days, and more than forty-one thousand people are killed or injured due to nodding off or falling asleep behind the wheel each year.

There's tons of research out there on the importance of sleep for health, how much sleep we need, the negative impact of sleep deprivation, and ways to get healthful, quality sleep. The truth is, not all the experts agree on the finer points regarding sleep—likely because every person is unique, with specific needs and health issues. Here's a short list of some of the generally agreed-upon negative health effects of sleep deprivation:

- Too little and too much sleep are both associated with hypertension, which in turn is related to heart attacks, heart failure, irregular heartbeat, and stroke.

- Sleep deprivation can lower your testosterone levels 10 to 15 percent, equivalent to a decade or more of aging, with concurrent reductions in libido, strength, ability to concentrate, and energy level.

- Reduced sleep promotes insulin resistance in people with type 1 diabetes as well as in healthy individuals. A lack of sleep is also a significant risk factor for the development of type 2 diabetes.

- Obesity and weight gain are also associated with sleep deprivation.

- Sleep deprivation has a negative effect on learning, memory, and overall cognitive function.

- The less you sleep, the worse your coordination and motor reflexes.

- Too little sleep can lead to elevated levels of inflammatory substances (e.g., interleukins, C-reactive protein) in the body, which can then lead to many inflammation- and metabolic-related conditions.

I don't want you to lose any more sleep over the details, but I do want you to consider these tips and guidelines on how to beat sleep deprivation and wake up feeling great:

- **Forget the rule.** The one about sleeping eight hours per night, that is. Just over seven hours (seven and a quarter to seven and a half) will do the trick, according to the experts. In a review of 1.1 million adults, researchers found that those who slept just over seven hours had less chance of dying after six years than those who slept more or less than that. In fact, the risk of dying was greater for those who slept more, not less. In addition, seven hours per night provides better cognitive performance than sleeping eight or more.

- **Invest in a red light.** Exposure to light during the night in any form—the television, your cell phone, a night-light, a laptop—can suppress the production of melatonin, the hormone that is responsible for keeping your sleep-wake cycle in sync. If you need to have some light to help you navigate to the bathroom during the night, make it red light.

- There are apps that will subtly **shift the tint and intensity of the light on your computer** based on the time of day; consider installing one if you're a computer user (and these days, who isn't?). It's not as good as unplugging completely, of course—but it's a pretty good solution.

- **Exercise early in the day.** Experts don't agree on how much time to keep between your workouts and bedtime, but the minimum is at least three hours. For the best shut-eye, exercise first thing in the morning.

- **Skip the alcohol.** Sure, a drink or two before bedtime may help you fall asleep, but it could also have you up and restless in a few hours, or you will be awake before your normal starting time, or both. The net result is restless sleep, and less sleep—not more.

- **Eliminate distractions.** That means you should keep the TV and computer off and your cell phone out of sight (if you need to have your phone in the room, keep it where you can't see it—and, if possible, put it on airplane mode so it's not receiving information). Once again, the light from these objects can reduce melatonin levels. If you fall asleep better with a little noise in the background, choose some soothing music or white sound.

- **Tame your alarm clock.** Hopefully someday you won't need this annoying object. If you don't need one now, great. If you do, don't use the snooze button. Discipline yourself to get up when it goes off. And if you can't, it's a pretty clear sign you need to get to bed earlier.

- **Be consistent.** Go to bed at the same time every night and get up at the same time every morning. That means Saturday and Sunday too! Work with your body's rhythms, not against them. I have this crazy timer in my body that puts me to bed at 10:24 p.m.

every night. Not 10:23 or 10:25. For some bizarre reason that's when I end up in bed, so I go with it.

- **Identify your magic bullet.** Okay, maybe it's not magic. However, if you have a routine you can do before bedtime that helps you fall asleep and stay asleep—perhaps it's meditation, a hot shower or epsom salts bath, doing crossword puzzles, reading, progressive relaxation—follow it consistently. But whatever you do, don't do it in bed. Take all the non-"S" activities out of bed, so your bedroom becomes a sanctuary for just sleep and sex, not work and watching TV.

- **Rethink naps.** A brief (ten- to twenty-minute) nap during the middle of the day can be helpful if you are really tired and feel like you will fall asleep at your desk or behind the wheel. However, a before-dinner nap can screw up your ability to fall asleep at your optimal time.

- **Have sex.** It's no secret that having sex can make you tired and also relieve stress. These are two essential ingredients for healthful sleep. For men, sex also releases a cocktail of hormones after an orgasm that promotes sleep, relaxation, and reduction of anxiety levels.

- **Don't fight it.** If you wake up during the night and can't fall back asleep within twenty to thirty minutes, don't get frustrated. Instead, choose to do something restful, such as reading, listening to soothing music, practicing deep breathing, or meditating. You should be ready to crawl back between the covers in no time.

YOU DON'T HAVE TEN THOUSAND HOURS

You've probably heard of Malcolm Gladwell's "ten thousand hours" rule, whereby the average amount of time spent by anyone who is said to have mastered a given skill is, yes, ten thousand hours.

It's a very appealing idea, which is part of why it's become so pervasive in our popular culture. Gladwell argues that time and passion—rather than talent and genetics—determine mastery, and, by extension, success in the world. It's a democratic idea. Anyone can succeed, he suggests. Hard work trumps talent.

Plenty of holes have been poked in Gladwell's theory since his book *Outliers* was published in 2008—chief among them that, while ten thousand hours is an average, the actual number of hours required to achieve mastery varies hugely from one individual to the next. Some people seem to require many tens of thousands of hours of diligent practice before they can approach mastery. Others, distressingly for us mere mortals, seem to stumble upon it almost by accident.

If you're an innate master of anything, good on you, and I imagine you're doing well for yourself. But even if we accept the claim that anyone can master anything in ten thousand hours, New Primers don't have ten thousand hours.

Think about it—ten thousand hours is:

Six hours a day,

five days a week,

forty-eight weeks a year,

for seven years.

Unless you're independently wealthy enough to forego gainful employment and can afford high-level lessons in your chosen endeavor for that entire period, forget about starting from zero at a completely new skill and mastering it before checkout time. It's unrealistic.

For years, I thought I'd eventually get around to learning to speak French or Italian. For a guy who travels a lot, that seemed like a reasonable goal to have, and I always admired the world traveler who could transition smoothly from one language to another. But recently I relieved myself of the burden of that obligation. I don't have the aptitude—or, more important, the passion—for it, and so I'm letting it go. My English (and my charming Australian manners) will have to suffice when I travel. For other people, learning a musical instrument is on their bucket list—but they're tone-deaf and they flunked music appreciation in grade school.

I'm not saying not to pursue new activities; just don't think you have to be a master of everything. Unlike the learning of foreign languages, flying is something I do have a feel for. My years driving high-performance sports cars, and the many hours I've spent on surfboards and skateboards, seem to have prepped me well for the unique demands of flight training and the dexterity it requires. I'm catching on, and, more important, I love it. I may never become Chuck Yeager, but I'll be good at it—and learning is its own reward.

I have also always wanted to be a faster runner, so I have taken up running with the California Coast Track Club, where alongside four-minute-milers, I'm trying to get better, stronger, faster. Not with the thought that I'll be Roger Bannister. Just with the thought that I'll be better.

The tone-deaf aspiring musician, similarly, might shoot for learning a few tunes on the ukulele rather than deciding he's going to be Eric Clapton.

We're obsessed with mastery in our culture—and with learning only as a means toward money, fame, power, and adulation. What if we pulled those ideas apart and said, let's learn for the pleasure of learning?

Many of us reach midlife and start trying to fit everything in that we feel we should have done—so we race toward the end, cramming all kinds of near-pointless activities into our already-overbooked lives. A better strategy is to choose judiciously, bringing to bear our own strengths, weaknesses, and temperaments on the question of how to spend our most precious—and least replaceable—commodity: time.

BRAINPOWER TIP #11: DO EVERYTHING ELSE IN THIS BOOK

My fiftieth year had come and gone.
I sat, a solitary man, in a crowded London shop.
An empty cup, an open book on the marble table top.
As on the shop and street I gazed,
My body of a sudden, blazed,
And twenty minutes, more or less,
It seemed so great, my happiness,
That I was blessed and could bless.

—W. B. YEATS, "VACILLATION"

This is my catchall, final exhortation in this chapter: build a healthy body to build a healthy mind. Your body and mind aren't separated. They're one thing. In many ways, taking care of your body *is* taking care of your mind. And vice versa.

That isn't just fanciful New Age speculation anymore. In recent years, science has demonstrated a connection between the length of a person's *telomeres*—the ends on chromosomes that resemble the pointy ends of shoelaces—and susceptibility to chronic disease and early aging. Telomeres (*TEEL-o-meers*) regulate a cell's ability to divide and reproduce itself properly. The longer the telomeres, the greater that cell's capacity to divide, and thereby replace itself in a healthy way. As telomeres shorten, the cells lose that capacity. They become genetically unstable, your tissues begin to die, and you become susceptible to chronic disease of all kinds, including dementia, Alzheimer's, and age-related synaptic decline. In essence, telomeres are slow-burning fuses, lit at birth, which, at one point or another, eventually burn down to the nub.

Sounds fatalistic, I know.

But hold on just a second. As it turns out, you can slow down the rate at which that fuse burns. And I bet you can guess how.

Exercise. Diet. Smart sleep practices. Meditation. Stress relief. It's all part of one big package, and your telomere length reflects all of it: the state of your mind *and* the state of your body. Victims of trauma and depression and mothers of chronically ill children, no less than people who live on junk food and never get up from the couch, lose telomere length faster than less-stressed people with better health habits.

So I'll leave you with that one final thought. If you pride yourself on your high-powered, big-time corporate lifestyle, and you think you can thrive in a seventy-hour-a-week pressure cooker by eating kale and putting in a few workouts a week, know that your telomeres know the difference. Your stressed-out lifestyle may well be doing just as much damage as if you were a Cheeto-stuffing couch potato.

But if you turn things around—lower your anxiety through meditation, clarify your goals, and reconsider how you deal with stress—your cells will respond accordingly. A pilot study by Dean Ornish found that just three months of smart self-care practices (including diet, activity, stress management, and social support) measurably increased telomere length. The less we spin out into regret over the past and anxiety about the future, and the more present we are to what's happening in front of us, the longer our telomeres tend to be—and therefore the sharper, happier, and healthier we are as well.

YOUR THIRTY-DAY ACTION PLAN FOR BETTER MENTAL HEALTH

1. **Rethink your midlife crisis.** Think of a crisis at this point in your life as a clear opportunity—and a personal invitation—to take action to clarify your direction.

2. **Carve out at least ten minutes a day of dream time.** You can't fix your life if you don't know what's wrong, and you can't go somewhere if you don't know where you're trying to go. Schedule time to contemplate these things.

3. **Rethink stress.** Stress in itself isn't necessarily bad. It's your body marshalling its forces. The more you recognize this, the healthier you will become.

4. **Cultivate friendships.** This month, connect with at least three male friends. Have a guy's night, play a sport together, grab beers (or club soda). If at all possible, get together in person. Call—don't email—one friend a day, for no other reason but to say "What's up?" And don't limit yourself to friends your own age: connect with former mentors, teachers, or students, young and old. If your current friends and social group are holding you back in life, then start looking for a new tribe.

5. **Meditate** at least ten minutes a day. You may want to do this before your ten minutes of dream time.

6. **Sleep** seven hours each night, going to bed and waking up at the same time every day.

7. **Create a goal ladder** detailing how you want to proceed with at least one of the bigger life goals you come up with. Then begin putting those practices into place.

CONCLUSION
When Lightning Strikes

When I was twenty-eight years old, I was struck by lightning.

That's not a metaphor.

I was out playing golf with my friend Geoff at a course on the eastern coast of Australia, where the weather—like just about everything else in that still-untamed country—can kill you. Unlike the occasional sprinkles we get in Southern California, storms in that part of the world come in hard, fast, and angry.

We were getting ready to tee off on the eighth hole when we noticed that the wind was starting to howl, the dark clouds were gathering, and the thunder was rolling in.

Then, just seconds after we had opened our metal-framed umbrellas to shield ourselves from the pelting rain, everything went black. Both of us instantly lost consciousness as a lightning bolt arced down, hitting the top of our umbrellas and striking us both.

We never even heard the thunderclap.

After some indeterminate period of time, we came to—and checked ourselves, frantically, for any sign of damage.

Incredibly, there wasn't any. We'd come through unscathed. Later, a friend who knows about these things theorized that if Geoff hadn't been with me to split the force of the lightning bolt, I would have been burnt to a crisp.

Lady luck was on my side.

Then again, brushes with death haven't exactly been uncommon in my life. A few years after the incident on the golf course, an ancient, one-hundred-foot pine tree bordering my property was struck by lightning (yes, lightning again). The tree fell and sliced through our house cleanly, destroying the room from which my wife had retrieved my youngest daughter just moments before.

Back in New Zealand, my nickname was "Just Miss"—for my otherworldly capacity to come through life-threatening encounters without a scratch. By some combination of foolhardy confidence, guts, and tons of luck, I somehow managed to make it through even the scariest of situations, body and soul intact.

Then there have been the other near misses in my life—split-second opportunities that have sprung up that I *have* leapt on and taken advantage of at just the right moment. Chances I recognized as enormously promising, but as fleeting as that flash of lightning. Chances that, ready or not, I had to seize in the moment and trust that I was smart enough and adaptable enough to figure out the details later.

As a near-homeless surfer kid in Australia with no experience in a kitchen beyond peeling potatoes and washing dishes, I talked my way into a head chef job—then worked hard enough to parlay that into similar jobs at many of the best restaurants in Queensland. I then set my sights on getting into university after studying sixteen hours a day and graduating in the top 2 percent in the state. A few years later, as a law student in need of extra cash, I talked my way (again) into a job at a brokerage firm—and became the first university student ever in Australian history to be licensed to trade stocks full-time.

I'm sure I've missed a few chances in my life, but I've tried to make it a habit to grab every lightning-strike opportunity I've received to reinvent myself many times over the years, from founding Australia's largest independent power company when I didn't know a kilowatt from a hole in the ground, to cofounding one of America's largest prepaid mobile phone companies when I barely understood how my own phone worked.

I've kept learning as I've gone along, grabbing opportunities on a hunch at every turn, right up to my latest endeavors in men's health—and now, this book.

I had no idea I could write a book, but I wanted to make it a part of my life's mission to help other men.

If there's a lesson for New Primers in all this, it's that *your life is yours to create, now and forever.* Wherever you are in your career, relationship, or finances, you can take the reins and reinvent your life for the better.

But jump while the jumping's good. When the passion and power and fire are there, dive in, full bore. Otherwise, the big revolutionary chance of a lifetime might pass you right by, and you'll never even hear the thunderclap.

Whether or not this has been your personal MO up to this point, it *can* be—and it should be. The happiest, most successful people in the current economy will be those who can move, adapt, change, and reinvent themselves. Not out of fear, but out of passion for something new, different, and better. The next revolution up the spiral staircase. The next evolution of you.

If I've done my job, this book will be the spark that ignites a new fire in you to make the changes you need to optimize your mental and physical health, so that you can dive into your next half century with new focus, vitality, and passion.

I wish you all the best—and much peace and happiness.

ACKNOWLEDGMENTS

CRAIG COOPER

I'm extremely fortunate to be surrounded by so many inspiring and successful people who have guided me in life, health, and business—and now with this book.

To Maria, my wife and love for thirty-five years. She has always been with me in sickness and in health as we pushed through all the challenges and opportunities in life together.

To my daughters, Montana and Lauren, who have endured my health and fitness obsessions over all the years. Hey, girls—Daddy now has a book to show for it!

Karen Rinaldi, my "surfer-girl" publisher at HarperCollins, who not only came up with the title of the book but was also a true partner, friend, and collaborator in every sense. Karen, what more can I say, you are awesome—let's do another one!

To Karen's extended team at HarperWave, including my fantastic editor, Sarah Murphy, who happily put up with my perpetual eleventh-hour edits, her editorial assistant, Hannah Robinson, and the rest of the Harper crew. So many of you to thank—you know who you are.

Of course, thanks to my agent and kindred spirit, David Black at the David Black Agency in NYC—who seems to get hit by a car every other year but keeps bouncing back like an eighteen-year-old. Dude, I am the last person to say "slow down," but at least look before you cross. I need you to stay healthy! Thanks for believing, D.

To Andrew Heffernan, my cowriter and friend. Thanks for all the long hours, research, advice, and passion that you brought to the subject matter. It was a great experience working with you. I realized very early into the project why our agents matched us up—they knew we would form a lifelong friendship beyond this book. Now get back to your own life, wife, and family!

Thanks also to the members of my extended health team, who have looked after me over recent years. Special thanks to my primary care physicians: Dr. Robert Huizenga, a rare doctor who is healthier, fitter, and more ripped than 99.999 percent of his patients—including me! Dr. Stuart ("Skip") Holden at Tower Urology (recently retired from UCLA). And my good friend and naturopathic guide, Dr. Geo Espinosa, at NYU Langone. To you all, I apologize for calling out the medical community in this book—you are absolutely not the intended targets. You are all passionate and caring educators. I am grateful to have you on my team.

Thanks also to my extended training crew and friends for inspiring and motivating me to keep pushing harder in life.

Thanks to all the trainers at Innovative Results in Costa Mesa, California—and especially Corey Beasley, who keeps me moving and injury-free (most of the time!). Thanks also to Corey for helping stage the mobility photos and for lending me your gym for the various multiday photo shoots.

My boxing trainers: John Snow at Trinity Boxing Club in New York City, and Shane Corbin at CDM Boxing in Corona Del Mar, California.

My running coach, Bill Sumner, from California Coast Track Club, for his energy and lifelong commitment to making us all faster.

To Gabby Reece and Laird Hamilton, for inviting me into your inner circle and allowing me to share in the passion and energy of your training sessions and life. You guys are an inspiration.

To Darin Olien, for being a great friend, training partner, and educator—you are a true and authentic messenger of clean and healthy living. The world is a better place with you in it.

And thanks to all my friends and training partners who continue to push the boundaries of peak performance as they age. Eric Hippeau, Gary Raugh, and Peter Grope, my sixty- and seventy-plus-year-old great friends and ski crew who still live life, charge, and ski powder like they were in their thirties. Every year you guys show me what is still possible in another ten to twenty years—so don't slow down!

And to Halister Brice for his advice, friendship, and personal counsel over the years, and for keeping me focused on what really matters in life—and helping me keep it all together.

Thanks also to all of you who contributed to the research involved with this book, including Deborah Mitchell and Amy Fox.

Thanks to Chris Tally at Precision Food Works for his valuable contributions on nutrition and natural testosterone therapy.

And to Robert Randall of Robert Randall Productions and Neil Kremer of Kremer Johnson Photography.

Finally, thank you to all the nurses who looked after me over all the months that I was in the hospital system in my preteen and teenage years. I have no idea who you are, but you guys and your counterparts all over the world are the true unsung heroes of the health care system.

Thanks to all of you. I am truly grateful.

Peace and health.

CRAIG COOPER
Newport Beach, California
May 2015

ANDREW HEFFERNAN

Thanks first of all to Craig Cooper for looping me in on this engrossing project. It was an honor and a pleasure to work with you on this Herculean task. Your passion for the topic was palpable every step of the way.

Much gratitude also to Karen Rinaldi, Sarah Murphy, and everyone at HarperCollins for their faith in me, and their support and encouragement throughout the whole adventure.

Thanks to David Larabell and Antonella Ianarinno at the David Black Agency for their diligence.

Thanks also to all my teachers, including Bill Hammond, John Lincoln, Tom Peyser, Michael Calabrese, Jane Ridley, Michael Connelly, Manuel Duque, Lisa Wolpe, Richard Warner, Bruce Gelfand, Elizabeth Beringer, and the many fitness professionals with whom I've had the honor of working over the years: Lou Schuler, Alwyn Cosgrove, Nick Tumminello, Angelo Poli, Shannon Turley, Jen Sinkler, John McGuire, Tony Gentilcore, the editors at *Men's Health* and *Experience Life*, and many others.

To my three favorite writers, James A. W. Heffernan, Nancy C. Heffernan, and Virginia Heffernan: thanks for all the inspiration, support, and wise words throughout my journey as a writer. The family trade got me too.

And finally, profound gratitude, admiration, and love for my wife, Heidi Rose Robbins, and our children, Kate and Dylan. You guys make everything worth it.

YOUR NEW PRIME
SHOPPING LIST

For more detailed shopping lists and specific product recommendations, go to www.thenewprime.com/shop.

FOODS

Organic/grass-fed/free-range should always be the priority when possible and where budget allows.
Where applicable, eat food in its raw state, not juiced.
No commercial fruit juices.
Frozen organic vegetables are okay.
Items marked with an asterisk are low on the glycemic index.

Meat and Dairy (always organic—and eat in accordance with Your New Prime guidelines in Chapter 3)

beef (*in very moderate amounts—see guidelines and look for organic, grass-fed only*)
butter (*organic, pasture-raised—look for a bright yellow color, indicating high omega-3 and carotene*)
chicken (*in moderation—see guidelines*)
eggs (*only pasture-fed/organic and free-range, maximum two servings a week*)
Greek yogurt (*organic, in moderation*)
kefir (*non-GMO, and use sparingly, as it is a dairy source*)

Seafood (use the "Seafood Watch" app to help purchase seafood from sustainable populations)

oysters
sardines (*only those in non-BPA cans*)
New Zealand mussels
wild Alaskan salmon (*Vital Choice brand offers home delivery*)
canned salmon and tuna (*BPA-free cans only*)

Vegetables

arugula
avocados
baby spinach
beets
bell peppers*
broccoli*
carrots

cauliflower*
green beans*
jalapeños
kale
lettuce (*boston, green leaf,
    red leaf*)*

mushrooms
onions (*red and white*)
parsley
sprouts
tomatoes (*raw or in bottles,
    never canned*)

Fruits

apples*
bananas
berries*
blueberries
cherries
grapefruit*

grapes
kiwis
lemons
limes
mango
olives

oranges
papaya
peaches*
pears*
pomegranates
watermelon

Grains and Cereals (*avoid gluten if intolerant*)

amaranth
barley
brown rice
buckwheat

couscous
kamut
oats and oatmeal
quinoa

wheat germ
whole wheat
Ezekiel-brand bread

Beans and Legumes

black beans
fava beans
garbanzo beans, hummus*

kidney beans
lentils (*green, red, and black*)
pinto beans

split peas
tempeh
white beans

Sweet Treats

dark 70–100 percent cacao
    chocolate (*cacao
    percentage depending
    on taste*)

dark-chocolate goji berries
dark-chocolate-covered
    almonds

Manuka honey
    (*from New Zealand*)

Nuts, Seeds, and Oils

almonds*

brazil nuts

cashews*

chia seeds

coconut oil

extra-virgin olive oil, cold-
pressed

flaxseeds and flaxseed oil

macadamia nuts

red palm oil

MCT oil

nut and seed butters (*e.g.,
almond butter, hemp
seed butter*)

palm kernel oil

pistachios

pumpkin seeds*

sesame seeds

sunflower seeds

walnuts

Grocery Items (*in glass jars or frozen, no cans*)

miso (*in moderation*)

pickles

sauerkraut

Herbs and Spices

cayenne

chili peppers

cinnamon

curry powder

garlic

ginger

turmeric

oregano

Protein Powders

Vega "Sport" Performance
Protein Powder

Paradise Herbs "Protein &
Greens" Vegan Protein
Powder

The "Dirty Dozen" and "Clean Fifteen"

Each year, the Environmental Working Group (EWG) prepares a list of the "Dirty Dozen," which is a list of the twelve conventionally grown fruits and vegetables that have the *most* pesticide residues. For 2014, the "dirty" list included apples, strawberries, grapes, celery, peaches, spinach, sweet bell peppers, imported nectarines, cucumbers, cherry tomatoes, imported snap peas, and potatoes. The number of different pesticides varies for each food item, but the concentrations are high relative to other produce. Always strive to buy only organic foods for those listed on the "dirty" list.

On the positive side, the EWG also prepares a list of the "Clean Fifteen." These fruits and vegetables have demonstrated few and low concentrations of pesticides. For 2014 they included avocados, sweet corn, pineapples, cabbage, frozen sweet peas, onions, asparagus, mangoes, papayas, kiwis, eggplant, grapefruit, cantaloupe, cauliflower, and sweet potatoes. "Clean" foods can be purchased nonorganic if your budget doesn't allow for the organic option.

Some Additional Prime Grocery-Shopping Rules

- Buy as much local produce as possible.

- Shop at local farmers markets.

- Avoid big organic brands (like Horizon milk, for example). Most large corporate organic brands are technically "organic" but fail many of my principles of healthy living (they use GMO seeds, have unhealthy living conditions for chickens, cows, and other animals, etc.).

- Buy eggs that come only from small nonfactory farms, and that come from chickens that are pasture-fed, free-range, and organic.

BEVERAGES

- coconut water

- organic coffee (*freshly ground preferred*)

- organic green tea

- organic hibiscus tea

- Japanese matcha "ceremonial" tea powder

- kombucha probiotic drink

- white tea

- almond milk

- rice milk

- coconut milk drink

- filtered water (*if buying in plastic bottles, avoid bottles with the recycling codes 3, 6, or 7*)

SUPPLEMENTS

Lots of supplements are recommended throughout Your New Prime. *Here are the main ones I take daily:*

vitamin D3 (*5,000 IU*)

omega-3 fatty acids

Prost-P10x (*for prostate health*)

EveryDay Male (*for sexual health*)

Men's Probiotic by PR Labs (*for gut health and immunity*)

cayenne

turmeric

modified citrus pectin

astragalus

CoQ10

magnesium L-threonate

ashwagandha

Cordyceps (*mushroom extracts*)

PERSONAL ITEMS

All must be labeled "fragrance-free" and contain natural oils. Visit www.ewg.org/skindeep/ for critical information about personal care products.

Deodorant: Make sure the type you choose is not aluminum-based (most that are labeled "antiperspirant" are; most with "deodorant" only on the label are not).

Soap: Avoid anything labeled "antibacterial." *Triclosan*, the chemical that kills bacteria, is a hormone disrupter currently on its way to being (rightfully) banned in commercial products.

Shampoo: Watch out for fragrances, preservatives, and the "surfactants" SLS, SLES, and DEA.

Mousse and gel: These products often contain carcinogens, human and animal toxicants, and environmental pollutants. Consider switching to an organic product.

Shaving cream: Anything that's as foamy and fragrant as the stuff your dad used to use is almost certain to contain nasty chemicals. Try using coconut oil.

Moisturizer and face creams: It's shocking how many chemicals we smear on our faces every day. Aim for chemical- and fragrance-free products.

Natural laundry products: Loaded with endocrine disrupters (often in the form of fragrances), laundry products are the most toxic personal care products on the market. Because we wear clothing covered with its residue during most of our daily lives, it also has a huge potential to do us harm. Detergents do not always list dangerous ingredients, so let the buyer beware on this one.

INDEX

ABOUT THE AUTHOR

Craig Cooper is a serial entrepreneur and health and wellness advocate for 40+ men's health. He is the founder of CooperativeHealth and Performance Research Labs and was the co-founder of the telecommunications company Boost Mobile USA. He holds dual degrees in law and economics from the University of Sydney and is a regular contributor to the *Huffington Post* on healthy aging. He lives in Newport Beach, California.